Meaningful Living across the Lifespan:

Occupation-based intervention strategies for occupational therapists and scientists

Meaningful Living across the Lifespan

Occupation-Based Intervention Strategies for Occupational Therapists and Scientists

Moses N Ikiugu and Nick Pollard

Whiting & Birch
MMXV

Published by Whiting & Birch Ltd,
Forest Hill, London SE23 3HZ

ISBN: (print) 9781861776365
ISBN: (ebook) 9781861770929

Contents

Contents

Acknowledgements

We would first and foremost like to thank all the reviewers who closely examined our book proposal and provided very useful feedback. Their comments helped make this book a much better product than it would otherwise have been.

Many thanks to David and the entire editorial team of Whiting & Birch Publishers, Ltd, for their assistance to us in this project.

Thanks also to our students, occupational therapy clients, and research participants in all our various scholarly ventures who continue to be our teachers and our motivators as we strive to be better clinicians, researchers, and teachers.

The first author would like to thank Marie Anne Ben for her love and support throughout this project, and Susanna Davila (his adopted mom) for her love, warmth, and support. As always, Susanna's pride in his work gives him strength to continue during those moments when he feels like giving up. Her feedback to an earlier draft of the book manuscript was very valuable.

The first author would like to thank his department Chair, Barbara Brockevelt, the dean of the School of Health Sciences, Mike Lawler, and the faculty in the Occupational Therapy Department at the University of South Dakota for their continued support in all his work. This book would not have been possible without all their support and encouragement.

Finally, he would like to thank his two children, Ivan and Nora, his sisters and brothers-in-law, and his nieces and nephews for always providing that critical family support that gives him the confidence to keep going in the knowledge that they are always available to support him in all he does, not matter what life brings his way.

The second author would like to thank his colleagues at Sheffield Hallam University for their support, encouragement and interest in this project, and Linda, Sally, Molly, Joshua, and Daisy for their patience when he was 'too busy working' for meaningful engagements.

Dedication

To my late adopted US dad, Dick Curtis who was a valued friend, mentor, and a gentle critic of all my work, and my adopted mom, Susanna Davila who continues to be a valuable source of love and support in all my work.

Moses

To my wife Linda, who makes it all possible

Nick

Introduction

Frankl (1992) postulated that the will to meaning is the primary motivation for behavior in human existence. Frustration of the pursuit for meaning, especially in the 20th century (and probably in the 21st century in the modern and Western world as well), constituted what he referred to as "existential vacuum". The cause of this vacuum is a decline of engagement in realistic transcendental activities such as philosophical discourses, religious practice, or activities providing a concrete sense of purpose such as planting and harvesting, combined with a corresponding increase in materialism, reductionism, and nihilism (Mascaro & Rosen, 2005). According to Frankl (1992), this existential vacuum led to a major disease of our times which he called "noogenic neurosis" (existential neurosis). Simply stated, noogenic neurosis may be conceptualized as a disease of meaninglessness. Symptoms of this 'disease', as Frankl termed it, include boredom, anxiety, alcohol and substance abuse, depression, and even suicide.

Although the medical implication of Frankl's description of noogenic neurosis as a disease might be debatable, his postulations have been discussed in detail by a host of psychologists, philosophers, and sociologists. Numerous studies have been conducted, and the results have been found to support these postulations. Chief among these findings is that there is a clear relationship between a sense of meaning in life and one's quality of life (Iwasaki, 2006), which strongly suggests a range of determining factors. Also, Frankl (1992) argued that while there was no universal definition of life meaning, some of its constituents included loving someone or something other than oneself, exercising choice of action (at least choice of attitude regarding how to respond to life events irrespective of circumstances), taking responsibility to solve problems presented by life and fulfilling requisite life tasks, and having a goal towards which to aspire (which may be perceived as a personal mission in life). In the rest of the book, we will refer to the problems identified by Frankl as "issues of meaning/meaningfulness/meaninglessness" rather than adopting Frankl's construct of "noogenic neurosis".

This departure from Frankl's terminology is necessary due to recognition of the fact that these issues are more socially based and therefore they are not 'diseases as such'. They are often consequences of social problems such as domination of minority by majority cultures with subsequent loss of indigenous cultural values, materialism that makes it very difficult for people to dwell on activities related to deeper reflection, self-understanding, meaningful connection with others, and meaningful connection to important institutions such as religious organizations or other bodies that provide guidance to individuals in formulation of values. Furthermore, people experiencing problems of meaninglessness are properly viewed as victims of these social dynamics. As such, we think it is wrong to refer to what they are experiencing as diseases because that would imply that they need to be cured, while what they really need is: 1) to learn how to cope with social problems; or 2) help removing social barriers to meaning in their lives.

Consistent with Frankl's discussion of the indicators of life meaning, based on factorial analysis, Iwasaki (2006) deduced some of the constituents of a meaningful life as: goal-oriented life, positive emotions, self-esteem, and sense of identity. According to Iwasaki, these factors have been found to be related to lower incidences of depression, high levels of hopefulness, and a good quality of life. It has also been found that positive emotions, self –esteem, sense of identity, and goal oriented life are enhanced through what occupational therapists and scientists refer to as occupations [i.e., "chunks of culturally and personally meaningful activity(ies) in which humans engage that can be named in the lexicon of the culture" (Clark, Parham, Carlson, Frank et al., 1991, p. 301)]. For example, participation in leisure occupations has been found to contribute to an experience of positive emotions and sense of well-being, positive identity and self-esteem, social and cultural connection, learning and development, and demonstration of personal strength and resilience, and in the process, to a sense of meaning in life (Iwasaki, 2006).

For a long time, work has also been recognized as a central constituent of a meaningful life. In the literary world, one of the best illustrations of this centrality of work to meaning-making is the story of Ivan Ilych (Bayley, 1967) written by Tolstoy (1960). In this story, Tolstoy described the desolation that Ivan Ilych, reflecting on his past life, felt at his deathbed. Having lived largely for the social and material benefits his position in the Ministry of Justice brought him, he suddenly realized how meaningless it had all been. In increasing physical pain he renounces everything, even his fear of death, and is finally able to die. As Michaelson (2007) observes in his commentary on the story, for many, work seems to be viewed as antithetical to meaningful life as seen in the statement that many people make to the effect that "one is too busy working" to be living (p. 335). Such statements, Michaelson argues, raise the question of whether working is the opposite of meaningful living. Illich (1980), for example, argued for the right to useful unemployment, and Lafargue (1996) for the right to be lazy. Clearly opinions about the meaningfulness of work are divided: some people argue that work has no meaning, and others argue that it is the essence of a meaningful life.

Michaelson further argues that the issue is not that Ilych or anyone else for that matter worked too much and therefore did not live as full a life as they might, or that the work they did was meaningless. Rather, the issue is that people fail "to live meaningfully" (p. 335). To avoid meaningless living, he suggests that one find a way of integrating work into his/her life such that it is part of "a life well lived" (p. 335). That means that one has to find a way of escaping the pitfalls of pathological use of work as illustrated in the apparently meaningless life of Tolstoy's Ivan Ilych. In the story, Ilych used his work as: 1) an escape from an unsatisfactory marital life, in which he uses the social and material benefits as a way of keeping his wife occupied and appeased; 2) a way to avoid facing the authentic self; 3) a way of avoiding confrontation with his bare humanity; and 4) his entire identity. Ilych thus failed to recognize the moral value of his work in terms of what it could contribute to the good of humanity, and therefore, it became essentially meaningless. However, if contextualized properly, work can be a deep source of meaning in one's life as illustrated by Frankl (1992). In a statement to a fellow prisoner at the Auschwitz concentration camp, Frankl passionately stated that the manuscript that he had smuggled into the camp at great risk to himself was his life's work. To him, this work contributed to his life meaning to the extent that he was ready to die for it precisely because he saw it as contributing to something larger than himself.

However, Frankl's life work was a creation, something in which he had invested himself and which represented the expression of his thoughts, i.e. it had a cultural dimension. Many people do not consider work to represent anything expressive. Rather, they see it as a means of earning money, although it may also be a source of opportunities for social interaction and expression of some interest. Lafargue (1996), Marx's son in law, wrote the Right to be Lazy in 1883 while living in Northern France. He was concerned about the conditions of workers in the textiles mills of the region, many of whom worked 14 hour shifts and were injured because they were so tired they were prone to accidents. The money they received was very low, and for all their long shifts and risk of injury or death, the goods they produced were often dumped on the market in order to be sold off quickly to make room for the newest textile fashions. Lafargue argued that the workers, many of them women and children, deserved better and safer conditions. Similar arguments are still raised with regard to the exploitation of children and other workers today in the manufacture of textiles, sports goods and fashion items. The factories which produce them have moved into countries where labor is cheap and guidelines for improvement of health and safety conditions are more relaxed. In the UK, the rising demand for low paid workers in the private agencies in the social care industry has resulted in many women working flexible hours but on low rates of pay. This often results in a noxious combination of low motivation and long shifts, with an increase in risks for back injuries and other forms of accidents and injuries. People who work in such conditions can hardly be seen as having an opportunity to see their work as having any meaning in their lives other than simply a source of money.

The contribution of the meaninglessness of work in the modern society to the problems that Frankl identified is clear. Illich (1980) argued that a lot of what was actually produced in a capitalist society was not assigned monetary value. The labor expended by people engaged in production of such goods, he argued, was therefore not recognized as having worth in capitalist terms, even though it was useful in helping to maintain community. For example, volunteering in a soup kitchen, caring for an elderly parent, or teaching kindergarten is not valued much in a capitalist economy. Yet, such work is critical to the well-being of the community and society as a whole, and therefore is very meaningful work in Frankl's sense. Furthermore, Illich maintained that many of the things produced in a capitalist system have a built in obsolescence, or else are subject to the manipulation of fashion. Therefore many workers are engaged in production of things which do not have real community value, such as producing 20 varieties of cereals, or 100 types of body-wash.

Many of the things we purchase with the money we earn from producing these things without real value are themselves without real purpose. We go shopping to buy things which make us temporarily feel good, but ultimately, they are not particularly useful. Clothes look good for a year or so and then become old fashioned. The average music CD or a DVD, once purchased, is probably played three times while in our possession and then never listened to or viewed again. Each year people in the UK generate tons of rubbish by buying things that they do not really need, and then find they have to get rid of. The same can be said of the US. All this garbage is stuff that other people make in their work, and that we buy with the proceeds of our work. As Ivan Ilyich (in Tolstoy's novel) finds out as he learns not to be so concerned about bent photograph frames or chipped new crockery, none of this matters very much. Illich (1980) suggests that a community held together by the voluntarily given work contributed by its participants might be more durable and healthier for its citizens than one characterized by accumulation of material things.

This view was reiterated by Putnam (2000) who pointed to one particular development which he thought was a source of the problem of decline in social capital (the value of other through our relationships with them) in the US as the fact that people invested so much of their energy in their work that they had no energy left to invest in their communities. He argued that work had become the community. However, because work itself was being redefined by a global economy in which job security was less guaranteed, the risk was that the work-based community was rootless and shifting. One day it was there and the next it was relocated to a place where labor and site costs were cheaper. Updike's Rabbit (1991a; 1991b) is perhaps an exemplar of this shift in community values and subsequent meaninglessness. In four novels the life of this character spans the transition from the pre-television age to an era of the proliferation of consumer goods progressing from athletic basketball jock to an overweight and flabby car salesman with a heart condition. At the end of the tetralogy he returns briefly to his youthful pre-occupation with basketball, but after a life of modern consumerism, this is a mere fancy. In his way, despite the possibility that his life has progressed downhill ever since the beginning of the narrative, Rabbit manages a similar last minute redemption as Ivan Ilyich, suggesting that even in the modern consumer-oriented society, redemption of a sense of meaning in peoples' lives is still possible.

Occupations, including those of leisure and work, offer powerful means through which individuals and societies can be used to mediate perceptions of meaninglessness and offer the redemption alluded to above. We can have confidence in the power of occupations in helping us achieve the above stated objective based on our observation that when people die, they are often remembered in terms of the things they did with other people, and mementoes related to such things as sports affiliations or social, usually family, roles. As we will see in chapter two, English worker-writers often defined themselves in terms of their work or other occupations, particularly occupations related to increasing a sense of personal efficacy and a feeling of connection to other people. It follows then that one way of addressing Frankl's problem of meaninglessness in modern society would be by helping people find ways of orchestrating their occupations in such a way that what they do every day helps them experience positive emotions, create a positive identity for themselves, connect to something bigger than themselves, love someone or something other than themselves. In the process of engaging in such occupations, people may experience a sense of well-being due to a feeling that their lives are meaningful and purposeful. A member of a gardening project in Sheffield described to Nick how attending an allotment group twice a week and being given a plant to grow and care for through the winter gave him something to structure his week, and a chance to connect to other people, which made that period of time very meaningful for him. Specifically, he stated:

> *I don't socialize with a lot of people outside the group and talk to anybody [...] it [taking care of the plant] does get me out of the house early in a morning and it does get me in a weekly routine. And that helps me a great deal, cause you wake up in a morning and you think 'Monday!, Ah I can go somewhere,' you start feeling you b*elong somewhere, *to me. And even later in the week, Thursday, I can go somewhere, even if I didn't have somewhere to go that's two days in the week I can have talks with people and possibly if I had a full weekly routine I wouldn't get a situation like this where I can talk to people like this, so this would still be beneficial no matter what situation.*

In their work, occupational therapists and occupational scientists can help people choose to engage in occupations that contribute not only to connection with other people, but also that facilitate connection to a cause that transcends personal "desires for pleasure or power" which would lead to "a meaning-saturated attitude" (Mascaro & Rosen, 2005, p. 987). By helping people create meaning in their lives through what they do as described above, occupational therapists and occupational scientists would be enabling them to develop personal and social strategies to resolve their perceptions of meaninglessness.

Furthermore, because occupational therapists and occupational scientists are educated to understand the form, function, and nature of occupations (Clark et al., 1991), it may seem that they are well placed to help people structure their occupational lives in such a way as to counter the experience of life as lacking meaning. Yet, there is little evidence that occupational therapists and scientists are proactively responding to this challenge to take their rightful place in serving humanity. That is perhaps why clients have repeatedly expressed disappointment with the services they receive from occupational therapists, while at the same time pointing out the potential of the profession to play a crucial role in helping people find meaning in their lives.

A good example of the above mentioned disappointment was by the world renowned astrophysicist Steven Hawking (1996), who wrote the following:

> Now, however, people with disabilities and other previously disadvantaged groups, such as women and blacks, are demanding that they should be able to play a full part in society. As I see it, your job as occupational therapists is to make sure that they can. *I cannot say that professional occupational therapists have been much help in my case, but may be I just did not encounter the right therapists.* (p. 27, emphasis mine).

Hawking went on to suggest that:

> With modern technology, it ought to be possible for many people with disabilities to lead a life in the community and to contribute to society. It is the task of occupational therapists to enable them to do this. The important jobs involve *mental and organizational abilities rather than physical strength and dexterity*. This is the direction in which people with disabilities should be encouraged rather than being put onto carpet making and basket weaving, *which are inappropriate for those who are mentally alive*. (p. 28, emphasis mine)

Occupational therapists need to respond to Hawking's criticism by de-emphasizing physical strengthening and focusing on helping people do things that make their lives meaningful. Although strengthening and re-education in motor functioning is indicated for some clients, these strategies should not be central to occupational therapy practice but only adjunctive to helping people engage in valued occupations. Criticisms similar to the one by Hawking have been leveled to occupational therapists by other famous clients, such as the eminent cultural and field anthropologist Robert Murphy (2001), who developed a spinal cord tumor in 1976 and described his experience in occupational therapy during his rehabilitation as a degrading, meaningless exercise.

If occupational therapists focus on helping their clients experience a meaningful existence by participating in society through engagement in valued occupations, they may answer Frankl's challenge to help people deal with the problem of meaninglessness resulting from an existential vacuum. In recent years, with the emergence of the new professional paradigm focusing on occupation-based, client-centered, and collaborative practice, meaningful occupations are being rediscovered as the foundational media for authentic occupational therapy practice (American Occupational Therapy Association [AOTA], 2014; Kielhofner, 2009). Numerous theoretical conceptual practice models have been developed to guide therapeutic interventions with meaningful occupational performance and participation in life as the overarching goal of therapy. Examples of such theoretical frameworks include the Model of Human Occupation [MOHO] (Kilehofner, 2009), Canadian Model of Occupational Performance (Law, Polatajko, Baptiste et al., 2002), and the Occupational Adaptation frame of reference (Schultz & Schkade, 1992; Schkade & Schultz, 1992; Cole & Tufano, 2008).

The notion of occupational meaningfulness and in particular how occupations are used in meaning-making has been explored extensively in the occupational science literature (Aguilar, Boerema, & Harrison, 2009; Hocking, 1994; Ikiugu, 2005; Kumar, 2010; Rozario, 1994; Shank & Cutchin, 2010). However, the constructs of life meaning, meaninglessness, meaningful occupation, etc. have not been clearly defined in the occupational therapy and occupational science literature. Similarly, the question of how individuals can be assisted to structure their occupational lives in order to enhance meaning in their lives has not been adequately answered. In order to meet the challenge posed by Hawking, Murphy, and others, we have to negotiate with people to facilitate their full access to participation and the pursuit of the important goals to which they aspire in their lives. Meaningful occupational performance may be one way of doing this.

Meaningful occupational performance is, as Seibers (2008) writes, a functional challenge especially for people with disabilities. For such people, meaningful occupational performance means

> living] with their disability, to come to know their body, to accept what it can do, and to keep doing what they can for as long as they can. (p. 69)

Initially Seibers' statement seems to be offensive, a point which he acknowledges. However, he goes on to explain that for people with disabilities to be properly represented in social discourse, they have to be recognized as who they really are, even as we recognize that the needs of every disabled person cannot be addressed, because there are neither the remedies nor the resources. If we recognize a need to mediate Frankl's problem of meaninglessness, we have to recognize that it is a problem which cuts across all demographics in a society which disables. The problem of meaninglessness in the sense suggested by Frankl is experienced by all people including those excluded from society due to disability. As Snyder and Mitchell (2006) point out, the basis of this exclusion is paradoxically located in the notion of individual equality. The idea inherent in the construct of equality is that we are all equal in this society. Unfortunately some are unable to participate fully because their disabilities prevent them from doing so. In that case, the answer is therapy and occupational therapy in particular.

Where does this leave occupational therapists? Perhaps a beginning point may be recognizing that while there is a range of technical skills, strategies, and interventions with which they can address the needs of people with disabilities, they (and all their multidisciplinary colleagues) may not have answers. Consequently, they have to navigate to a solution by working with their clients rather than patronizing them. This denotes that client-centeredness has to be critically explored as a way for occupational therapists as professionals to work in collaboration with their clients to optimize availability of resources to enable clients participate fully in society. If they are to employ a concept like meaningful occupation, occupational therapists have to be clear about what they mean by meaningfulness. An attempt will be made to explore this construct from multiple perspectives in the rest of this book.

Organization of the book

The book can be conceptualized as consisting of four parts:

1. Foundational knowledge about meaningfulness/meaninglessness;
2. The role of occupations in meaning-making;
3. Guidelines for action to facilitate meaning-making through occupational performance; and
4. Thoughts about the future of occupational therapy and occupational science in helping people construct meaningful lives by contributing to the solution of pressing global issues through occupation-based initiatives.

To navigate towards a solution of meaninglessness in peoples' lives, occupational therapists must also develop a useful framework that they can use to guide their clients in meaning-making through occupational performance. This book is designed to contribute towards meeting these objectives. Its purpose is to help occupational therapists and occupational scientists think of new ways of applying their knowledge of the nature, form, and function of occupation to help all people, not only the sick and disabled, develop strategies to overcome their existential vacuum and in the process, resolve either the problem of meaninglessness in their lives or recognize and begin to address the social origins of the experience of meaninglessness. It is hoped that this book will offer occupational therapists and occupational scientists useful guidelines that they can use to be effective consultants in helping people orchestrate daily occupations in such a way that their work, self-care, and leisure occupations contribute towards an experience of positive emotions, creation of positive identities, connection to something larger than themselves, and ultimately towards experiences of life as optimally meaningful.

Part 1

In chapter one, we examine the definition of meaningfulness from multiple perspectives. The purpose of the chapter is to help clarify what the constructs meaningfulness and meaninglessness precisely mean, so that as therapists using the book help people organize their occupations to enhance meaning in their lives, they are able to identify indicators of meaningfulness that they can use to measure the effectiveness of chosen strategies.

However, an intellectual definition of meaningfulness is not enough. It is important to find out what people perceive to be meaningful in their lives. To achieve that objective, we analyzed autobiographies published by a community of "worker writers" in England using heuristic interpretive methods, with a view to teasing out what these individuals perceived to be the meaning of their lives and how they saw their daily occupations contributing to that meaning. Our findings of the analysis are reported in chapter 2. By understanding the experienced phenomenon of meaningfulness/meaninglessness as described by "worker writers", we set the stage in this chapter for the content discussed in subsequent chapters.

Based on Frankl's (1992) postulation that meaning in life derives from love for someone or something, creative activity, appreciation of beauty and art, connection to something larger than ourselves, and moral integrity, in chapter three, we embark on an exploration of how human beings have gone about, through the ages, searching for meaning in their lives. Frankl suggested that part of the cause of the existential vacuum in our times was disconnection from the natural environment and from traditions, including religious practices. Therefore, in chapter three we examine how culture and social norms, religion, and philosophical and scientific inquiry, are used by many people as vessels to convey them to an experience of meaning in their lives. This theme is continued in chapter four where we examine how occupations fit into meaning-making endeavors by grounding one in culture, religion, and social life.

Part 2

In the second part of the book (consisting of chapter 5), we explore the notion of occupations as media for meaning-making in life. We bring all the constructs discussed in the book together by examining how occupations are used as means of meaning-making by helping people develop the needed skills and accomplish developmental tasks at each stage of life. We also discuss how these occupations are grounded in the vehicles of meaning (culture, religion, social life, and philosophical/scientific inquiry) as discussed in chapter 3.

Part 3

In the third part of the book, consisting of chapter 6, we present a framework that can be used to guide individuals in structuring their occupations so as to optimize the sense of meaning in their lives.

Part 4

Finally, in the last part of the book consisting of chapter 7, we conclude our discourse with an examination of how major global issues such as climate change, poverty, and material inequalities are not only caused by human occupational performance, but also can be resolved through change in such performance. We argue that occupational scientists and therapists can broaden their scope of influence by finding occupation-based solutions to these issues. This can be achieved by helping people achieve optimum meaning in their lives by changing their occupational behavior in such a way as to contribute to amelioration of these issues, and in the process to experience themselves as contributing to a cause that is larger then them (in the process, helping them achieve a sense of transcendence through occupational performance).

Introductory case

Sarah is 38 years old, married, and she and her husband have 3 children. She is a college professor by profession. Her worker and mother roles take most of her time. For leisure, she likes to exercise, particularly running. She competes annually in the marathon and thinks that running is good for her physical and mental health, enhances her productivity at work, and gives her energy to take care of her children. Her religious faith is also a big part of her life. She says that attending church every week and engaging in activities to foster her faith, and to bring up her children according to church teachings are all very important activities for her. She enjoys watching sports, participating in outdoor activities, and maintaining connections with her extended family.

Sarah states that what gives her life meaning includes: participating in marathon competition; being a good mother and wife; attending church and engaging in other religious activities; watching sports on TV; engaging in outdoor activities; maintaining contact with her extended family; and having a meaningful career that gives her a feeling that she is doing something worthwhile with her life. She feels that because she is able to engage in all the above occupations, she experiences her life as meaningful, and that everything that she is doing has a purpose or a meaning behind it. She sums up her perception of what gives her life meaning as follows:

> I think that comes back to whatever I am doing, that I am giving everything that I have to it, that I am putting my best effort into whatever I am doing. It comes back to faith because that's one of the ways that I demonstrate what my God wants me… that's how I demonstrate that his love for us is to do everything in our day for him.

Sarah creates meaning in her life by: engaging in leisure occupations that make her feel **competent** (competing in the marathon); participating in activities that facilitate **connection** with other people including extended family; loving her family; **connecting to a reality that is larger than her** (her religious faith), and engaging in a profession in which she feel that whatever she does is **worthwhile**, that she makes a difference in peoples' lives. All the above are postulated by Viktor Frankl (1992) as criteria for a meaningful life. In this book, we will use Frankl's principles as outlined in logotherapy to examine how people can be guided to use their daily occupations to make their lives meaningful just like Sarah's life as described above.

In addition, because this book is about using occupations in new ways to enhance health and well-being for all people (not just those who have clinical diagnoses), in the final chapter, we offer our thoughts regarding the direction in which occupational science and occupational therapy can go in order to contribute more broadly to addressing broad social concerns. We hope that the ideas presented in this chapter will encourage debate in the profession of occupational therapy and the discipline of occupational science regarding how to join other scientific disciplines in engaging the population to solve major social challenges of our times.

PART I FOUNDATIONAL INFORMATION

In this part of the book, the groundwork is laid for use of daily occupations as a meaning-making tool in life. In chapter 1, Frankl's (1992) claim that existential vacuum and a sense of meaninglessness are the primary problems of the contemporary society are examined. His assertion that meaning-making is the anti-dote to the problem of meaninglessness irrespective of one's life circumstances is introduced as the rationale for the book. An attempt is made to define meaning from the philosophical and spiritual perspectives. The objective understanding of meaning is compared and contrasted with the subjective view of the construct. A working definition pertaining to the role of every-day experiences as the material from which meaning is constructed is generated.

In chapter 2, the working definition of meaning is verified through an analysis of the experiences of English worker-writers as expressed in their autobiographies. These experiences are used to ground understanding of the construct of meaning in life. In chapter 3, the human search for meaning is metaphorically compared to a journey or quest. Belief supporting institutions (including cultural and religious beliefs and cultural imagination as expressed in folklore, myths, and legends), and intellectual activities through philosophical discourse and scientific inquiry are examined as vehicles that are used by human beings in their journey in search for meaning.

In chapter 4, the sources of meaning in this human quest are identified as establishment of emotionally intense relationships, engagement in work and leisure activities, and adherence to idea systems. The dimensions of meaning in this journey are identified as establishment of a sense of self-worth, a sense of purpose in life, a sense of control irrespective of one's circumstances in life, and ability to express personal values. The four chapters in part I of the book are intended to prepare the reader for part II in which the way in which occupations are used in conjunction with each of the three sources and four dimensions of meaning at each developmental stage to facilitate a sense of purpose and meaning in life is discussed.

Chapter 1 Developing a working definition of meaningfulness

Learning objectives

After reading this chapter, the reader will understand:

1. Viktor Frankl's notion of human search for meaning and the hypothesis that daily occupations can influence one's sense of meaning in life
2. How meaningfulness can be viewed from a variety of perspectives:
   - Philosophical
   - Spiritual
   - Objective versus subjective
3. Criticisms that can be leveled against each view of meaningfulness
4. A working definition of meaningfulness that will be used throughout this book

Contents of this Chapter

- Meaning and social context: an overview
- Quest for meaning, spirituality, and the influence of changing environmental and social contexts
- Evolution of meaning through human history
- The big questions about meaning: multiple perspectives – philosophical, spiritual, psychological, sociological
- A working definition of meaningfulness/meaninglessness

Introduction

For much of human history the experience of a large majority of ordinary people was that life was often precarious, influenced by the fluctuations of war, famine, or the spread of diseases (Fernandez-Armesto, 2001). The advent of industrialization which brought people from agricultural communities to the urban centers in Europe and America often exposed people to new health risks or produced sordid living conditions in which life expectancy actually fell[1]. For example, people employed to grind blades in the cutlery trade in Sheffield, United Kingdom often died from lung diseases when they were still in their twenties due to the dust that they inhaled while at work. Cholera, typhoid, and tuberculosis often resulted from people living in overcrowded, poorly maintained environments. Poor housing, diseases, as well as high female and childhood mortality rates created the impetus for the development of the nascent caring professions in the late 1800s: nursing, social work, midwifery, and, by the early 1900s, occupational therapy. Although the thesis in this book is that daily occupations, including work, leisure, and self-care can be used as sources of meaning in peoples' lives, the argument that work is a source of meaning may be challenged given the poor conditions in which many of the workers still live today. In the 1900s, for many people, the building of cities offered different ways of surviving and defined an existence that was in contradiction to the philosophy of work. Large numbers of city inhabitants were involved in criminal activities, and an underworld culture of alternative values expressed in the language of that context developed. The resulting social differences between the mainstream culture and the underworld still remain important today (Linebaugh, 1991).

Victor Frankl

Before making any attempt to explore how various daily occupations can be used in meaning-making, in this chapter we will discuss in general the notion of meaning itself. In this regard, we begin with an examination of the work of Viktor Frankl. This charismatic psychotherapist became known for his work on the meaning of human life. He began working as a youth counsellor and as a doctor in the 1920s in a Viennese hospital department that catered for women suicide survivors. His experiences, and particularly those under the Nazi regime while he was living in the Theresienstadt ghetto and then during a period of incarceration in a series of concentration camps, became the basis for his work on the human search for meaning as the major motivator in life. These ideas led to the development of logotherapy, an intervention designed to combat meaninglessness and nihilism. According to Pytell (2007, 2000), Frankl's first book was dictated in 9 days, yet the uplifting messages it contained turned it into a best seller. **Frankl's story was that he survived the horrors of the Nazi concentration camps because he had something to look forward to, a goal for which to survive.** Consequently, in logotherapy, he suggested that humankind can overcome its worst fears (as he did) if only 'each of us does his best' to pursue a worthy goal in life (Frankl, 1992, p. 154). This is the basis for our recommendation in chapter 7 that people articulate personal mission statements clearly, so that these personal missions in life can be the basis for establishment of worthwhile goals to pursue in life, leading to a meaningful existence.

Criticism of Frankl

Frankl grew up in a comfortable Viennese Jewish family and had been educated as a doctor. Initially he was a follower of Freud's psychoanalytic tradition, and later of Adler's teachings. Even though he could have escaped the holocaust altogether, he found himself remaining in Nazi Austria to look after his parents at the beginning of the war. Pytell (2007, 2001, 2000) asserted that Frankl survived by co-operating with the Nazis in experimenting on the brains of Jewish suicide victims, activities in which his peers refused to engage. He was later confined in the concentration camps where he worked as a doctor. Pytell (2007) noted that it may be unreasonable to criticize Frankl's actions in the hindsight of an historical perspective gained in times of peace, considering that these were the actions of a person trying to survive under extremely terrifying circumstances.

Nonetheless, the reader is cautioned to bear in mind that the personal story Frankl frequently told could be selective and misleading, although as it remains without doubt the story of a holocaust survivor, it contains meaning and truth. Pytell (2000) suggests that Frankl's work likely dramatizes his survival, representing his own rather than 'Man's' cry (Frankl, 1992) for meaning, an unheard cry at that (Frankl, 1978). None the less, Frankl's (2000, 1978, 1969) writings gained wide acceptance over time, especially his observation that the contemporary society was sick due to the loss of meaning in people's lives. He referred to this condition of meaninglessness as *noogenic neurosis*. He described it as an existential vacuum resulting from a loss of touch with the natural environment; loss of grounding in traditions, religious practices, and philosophy; and the lack of a self-transcendent connection to something larger than ourselves. Symptoms of the malady were boredom and meaninglessness which were expressed through aggression, addiction, depression and suicide (Frankl 1992, 1969).

In this book, we use Frankl's notion that human beings are primarily motivated by a search for meaning in life. We agree that a lack of meaning in life can plunge one into a sense of emptiness (Frankl's 'existential vacuum') and subsequently into a lack of a sense of well-being. This lack can in turn lead to self-destructive behaviors such as addictions and even suicide. However, rather than subscribe to Frankl's pathologization of meaninglessness as a disease, we prefer to follow Maslow's (1970) suggestion that the search for meaning is actually a search for personal growth. We then propose that occupational therapists and scientists can help people realize this search for growth and ultimately for meaning in life by enabling them to carefully select occupations in which they participate every day of their lives.

Frankl's ideas as a guide to meaning-making

Our discussion of Frankl's theory is consistent with McNamee's (2007) suggestion that: 'Human beings are meaning junkies. It is not enough for people to just experience the world as it is; we are desperate to make sense of it' (p.1 of 15). However, McNamee's perspective of 'meaningfulness' is not existential, but seems to belong to a Western middle class understanding of life meaning found in the puritan values of hard work and healthy leisure which evolved over the 19th century (Flanders 2006; James, 2006). The dominance of this perspective of meaning originated from the growth of the middle classes during the 19th and 20th centuries, when there was a demand for a variety of professional occupations consistent with a rapid economic development. Such professional disciplines included engineering, teaching, medicine, and banking among others. The professionals defined themselves by their work, and were eager to distinguish themselves from the laboring classes in the neighbouring streets. These distinctions were based on a range of values: cultural, spiritual, educational, and familial. They were visible in the evident disparities in health between the wealthy and the poor.

The poor were very often held to blame for their own condition. Eugenic ideas of natural fitness and unfitness for genetic survival were used to spread fear that the healthy and wealthy might be contaminated by the rising numbers of diseased and impoverished people (James, 2006, Werskey, 1994). During that time in Britain, a third of the population was barely able to feed itself properly (Marr, 2009; Werskey, 1994). Even today, while there have been overall improvements in health, significant differences in life expectancy – between 71 for men and 78 for women in Glasgow compared to 85 for men and 87 for women in Chelsea and Kensington - remain the same as they were in the 1930s (National Records of Scotland 2011; Thomas, Dorling, & Smith, 2010). These disparities are still held to be natural [and perhaps pre-ordained] (Dorling, 2011). Under these circumstances of gross disparities, many working class people related 'meaning' to the value of their experiences and their place as witnesses to history. Their perceptions of quality of life were recorded in written autobiographies (Ragon 1986; Vincent 1981) as well as in folk songs (Buchan, 1997; Copper, 1975; Lloyd, 1969).

Thus, even within a particular culture the search for meaning can represent different things for different people. For those in the upper socio-economic status, meaning is perceived differently in comparison to the understanding by those in the lower socio-economic ranks. Even Frankl (2000, 1992, 1969) acknowledged that there is no one universal definition of the construct of meaningfulness. Rather, meaning is embedded in the concrete engagement in tasks that help individuals achieve specific goals, particularly **transcendental missions in life, or to create desired legacies which are intended to continue once their lives are over** (Frankl, 1969).

One complication when considering how people maintain a meaningful existence in the modern world is that technological gains appear to have eliminated many of the evolutionary challenges which gave meaning and purpose to life. For example, people no longer need to walk because they can get around by driving; they don't need to climb stairs because they can use a lift; and they do not even need to retain and recall information because they can access the internet through their phones. Many tasks that in the past made people feel competent (one of the ways in which people experience meaning in life) have disappeared. Instead of dealing with the challenges of survival, the problem facing the modern human being has become the question of what to survive for. The paradox is that people have an unprecedented ability to survive and to stay alive even in cases of severe injury or illness, but have 'nothing to live for' (Frankl, 1978, p. 21).

Creating meaning and happiness by not actually pursuing either

Throughout history, the nature of human action was often determined by social and cultural factors that ensured that achievements were recognized by an individual's peers and often more significantly, met the demands of the gods. Frankl (2000) argued that these motivations for action were always present even if they were not always recognized. The way to address the urge to achieve was to desist from merely striving to win for the sake of winning, for happiness, or for other gains. Striving to achieve happiness often led to loss of happiness. Such efforts resulted in aggression and were often unsuccessful. A better attitude in life, he suggested, was to adopt a philosophy of doing one's best while paradoxically maintaining self-detachment. Success and happiness would naturally follow (Frankl, 1978). He described a 'will to meaning' (p. 15) as a determination to achieve an end despite everything that may stand in the way of one's objective. He frequently referred to the idea of heroism which he argued pertained to finding meaning even in suffering (Frankl, 1978, 1969), making it possible to rise above pessimism and fatalism in the face of the inevitability of failure or death. If individuals could recognize that their past achievements could not be taken away from them, they could gain a sense of value, purpose, and meaning, and realize the potential for change, despite death or loss.

In occupational therapy, do Rozario (1994, p. 46) agreed with Frankl's position by asserting that the profound 'human longing for ritual and meaning' was expressed through spiritual pursuits. It is important to point out though that forms of spirituality may have actually originated from practical concerns about the necessity to organize society and to structure communal tasks in order to ensure human survival in particular environments (Mair, 1962; Pryor, 2004). Spirituality thus became important in imbuing humanity with a sense of meaning, yet also served to both uphold and sometimes challenge the status quo throughout the development of human societies. However, though people subscribed to religious beliefs, they tended not to be involved with the deeper discussion of the significance of such beliefs. Such discussion occurred amongst intellectuals concerned with sacred discourses (Berger, 1973).

Frankl's writings link the quest for human meaning with spirituality and imply that the spiritual crisis of meaning is rather a modern phenomenon. These views appear consistent with a wider recognition of the effects of loss of spirituality and the ritual that comes with it. For example Marr (2009, p. xi) and Dorling (2011, p. 24) suggest that a feature of modern society is that people have abandoned a purposeful [spiritual] ideology and are 'shopping' for new guides to a deeper significance to their lives, be it popular astrology, feng shui, angels, crystal therapy or Mayan prophecy (Redfield, 1994). Many of the traditional religions have also at times been rejuvenated to become part of the spiritual bazaar of our times (Berger, 1973).

The development of meaning

In his exploration of a history of truth, Fernandez-Armesto (2001) suggested that the initial ways in which humans understood the world around them was through the senses and the interpretation of feelings and emotions. In her analysis of African social systems during the early to mid-20th century, Mair (1962) extended this notion of meaning through interpretation of experiences by describing how social and political relationships were determined by the resources (that provide environmental experiences) available to particular communities. The development of communal ways of living, the use of ritual to mark key events in these societies and the systems of government necessary for distribution of goods and to ensure social survival were all determined by what was available to the people in the environment around them. Mair's analysis supports Wilcock's (2006) suggestion that the nature of human occupation, doing, being, becoming and belonging, is determined by the way in which the environment itself is occupied.

These commentaries suggest that many aspects of the meaning of human life are rooted in the everyday and ordinary, as they are encapsulated in the environment and the resources that it affords, than the pursuit of profundity. Putnam's (2000) discussion of social capital, for example, suggests that the introduction of television in the last century replaced communal activities with a form of entertainment which encouraged social isolation. The invention of television marked a significant stage in human development. The television itself depended on access to a wide range of resources in order to manufacture the complex components of the device from raw materials. The effect of television, however, was compounded by the dislocation of places of work from the community. The production of commodities such as the television required large scale and specialized industries needed to manufacture the components, and these factories required larger forms of organization and infrastructure such as transport networks. Small communities no longer offered adequate resources to support the growing population of people involved in these industries. Cities and towns grew and people increasingly commuted to work. The effect of introduction of the television was similar to that of the train earlier. In both cases, the production of affordable material commodities impacted on the nature of human occupation.

Prior to the onset of rapid urbanization, people shared in communal sports, talked together on the front porch, attended activities together, and thus formed part of the fabric of a socially engaged way of life. Putnam (2000) contended that it was through these activities that people recognized each other as members of the same community. The spread of television entertainment marked the point where this form of community ceased to exist in many parts of modern America and elsewhere in the world. Today, Putman observes, people invest more time with friends at work and home has become just a dormitory-like facility in the suburbs which only serves as a place to sleep. They have little to do with the locales in which they live, and the urban planning of communities reflects this altered way of life.

However, there are some grounds for skepticism about this view. One of the iconic examples of urban planning in the UK, which is an example of the separation of home from work, is the new city of Milton Keynes. Much of the vilification of this city and the many post war towns or urban developments which arose in the post war period, such as Stevenage, Crawley, or Swindon, has tended to be based in a form of snobbery rather than an examination of the quality of the lives of people there. To be sure there are people who live in social isolation in badly planned housing developments, but a sense of community, and therefore of the meaning associated with these developments is often evident (Clapson, 2004).

Other criticism comes from the strong indications of nostalgia for the lost sense of community and its supporting environment in modern times, combined with some rebellion against the nature and content of popular culture. The growth of industrial society produced overcrowding and filthy living conditions necessitated by poverty in many Western urban communities (Brogan, 1990; Foner, 1980, 1965; Marr, 2009; Zeldin, 1979). Marr (2009) among others noted that the forms of popular culture which arose from the 19th century urbanization and resulting squalor, while being adopted by the rising middle classes, were none the less often despised for the vulgarity which derived from their familiarity with every aspect of human life. The content of this popular culture was often sentimental, sometimes focusing on religious themes, sometimes subservient to the status quo, perhaps mindful not to go foul of the wealthier patrons in society (Russell, 1997). In order to be made attractive to the dominant view, the contents of this popular culture were often cleaned up or their meanings obscured (Lloyd, 1969).

The squalid conditions described above generated social pressures leading to a series of housing reforms, the development of affordable public housing, and culminating in the new towns and cities of the late 20th century. Some people in the communities resulting from these housing schemes developed aspirational values as suggested by Clapson's description of Milton Keynes image of 'Middle England' (2004). People who moved to these homes left their overcrowded environments and streets behind, and yet some looked back to the familiar community feeling this close proximity with others afforded. The mixture of sentiments this ambivalence suggests may be one of the reasons that the meaning that any culture confers to human life has become contested. Some aspects of culture become sanitized or suppressed in order to be palatable to the majority view in society. Further, the hardships of the past can become romanticized in historical re-interpretations of cultural experiences (Bromley 1989). If this is so, to what extent does cultural content accurately represent the meaning of the lived experiences of those who live the life that it is supposed to represent?

Another consideration as we attempt to understand how the whole notion of 'meaning' in human life develops is the observation that meaning appears to be historically intertwined with the development of spirituality, although this may depend on the nature of belief, which is a social construction. For much of the western world, spirituality seems to be connected with the rise and development of the church and the culture of Christianity, particularly in relation to the church as an institution through which religious meaning is interpreted and managed. According to Berger (1973) one of the purposes of religion was to provide a mechanism through which a consistency of meaning could be achieved. For a long period of time in the European history, Christian religion had been a key institution that structured the relationships between people, their rulers, and the stability of the world around them. However, many folk customs derived from earlier belief systems and these were frequently accommodated in the rituals and practices of the church, particularly in Western Europe. St. Patrick and St. Columba for example had to make their arguments for their faith using the language of their hostile druidic or bardic adversaries. The church itself preserved the ancient celtic cultures of Brittany (Markale, 1977) and Ireland (Lydon, 1998; Nagy, 1997) and, some argue, a form of the druidic tonsure (Ellis, 1994). These were ways of both asserting new spiritual meanings, and accommodating something of the old ways which people were being asked to give up. This kind of incorporation often appears to have taken place, although it does not always occur, in the adoption of new religions.

In order for those who professed the new religion to communicate its purpose, they had to accept elements of the indigenous cultures. For example, the 19th century British missionaries to China were encouraged to adopt Chinese dress and customs (Worrall, 1988). Often the church had to address the everyday needs of the people as a part of enabling them to find meaning in the Christian religious faith. During the rise of industrialisation, the English church and its various denominations launched missionary initiatives geared towards addressing the needs of the rising numbers of poor and oppressed groups of people, who were disadvantaged by the rapid social changes. These included initiatives to increase literacy to promote Bible reading as a way of encouraging church attendance (Edwards, 1984; Worrall 1988). These efforts of the church to create meaning in people's lives did not eliminate class tensions. The middle class quest for meaning included both a desire for social distinction from the poor, whom they saw as lesser beings and as objects for social reform (James, 2006; Marr, 2007, 2009). They felt guilty about depending on the labor of the working class poor for their bourgeois comfort, while at the same time they attempted to contain the threat posed by the animalistic atavism social reformers such as Seebohm Rowntree or Charles Booth perceived to be perpetuated by the savagery of these poor (Marr, 2009).

The society in the 19th century was partly characterized by a rising middle class, with greater opportunities for men to travel, or perhaps work in the colonies. This development led to increasing numbers of middle class women with no prospect of marrying unless they did so below their social class. Others perhaps found that with the general level of ignorance of sexual matters and rising number of cases of venereal diseases, marriage was not a good prospect (Marr, 2009). These women were trying to find something purposeful to do at a time when disparities and consequent social injustices were increasing with population growth and migration. What came out of these social dynamics were in part the development of Christian socialism and the growth of evangelical religious movements (Jones, 1984) in which some of these women became involved. This was the context within which a number of key health and social care professions such as nursing, social work and subsequently occupational therapy were developed (Frank & Zemke, 2008; James, 2006; Pearsall, 1983; Pollard & Walsh, 2000; Sakellariou & Pollard, 2008; Trollope, 1994). These emerging professions gave women career structures which were unavailable elsewhere in strongly male ordered societies (Frank, 1992). Thus, a continuing theme of the pursuit of life meaning was that people in the working class aspired to the values of the dominant middle class culture (Haylett, 2003; James, 2006), and these aspirations began with middle class attempts to find meaning for themselves in response to changing social circumstances. While the social inequalities of the 19th and early 20th century were an important part of the context which gave birth to a range of health and social care professions, it is ironically possible that the economic problems of the first decade of this century generated a depletion of resources in the public sector affecting many of these health and social care workers and a resurgence of similar injustices (Dorling, 2011).

A perennial search for meaning

Frankl's (1992) diagnosis of a social illness of meaninglessness may be appealing to those who are sensitive to the unjust consequences of economic changes, but the search for meaning by human beings involves much broader questions. Adams (1979, p. 125) points out that of the 'problems connected with life [...] some of the most popular are: Why are people born? Why do they die?' Most people will have considered questions of this nature at various points in their lives. The search for meaning is a perennial human quest, and therefore should be a concern for occupational therapists and occupational scientists as part of their consideration of holism, client centeredness, meaningful and purposeful doing, and human functioning in relation to the environment. Occupational therapists in particular need to facilitate the process of answering these questions by their clients in order to optimize meaningful living. Frankl's promotion of hope through transcendentalism provides the kinds of answers that would be available in religion. In this chapter, meaningfulness will be discussed as it has been defined by philosophers, psychologists, sociologists, theologians, and scholars from other disciplines. This definition will be a basis for exploring in subsequent chapters: how human beings have gone about searching for meaning throughout history; and how they can learn to live meaningfully through what they do (their occupations) every day of their lives.

About meaning

Philosophical definition

In the first section of this chapter, we made the point that human beings are, and always have been in search for meaning in their lives, and this search has always been connected to the development of society, culture, and community. In this section, we will go further and try to clarify what we mean by 'meaning', 'meaningfulness', and 'meaninglessness'. At the outset, it is important to point out that the notion of meaning is a vague construct. As the authors have repeatedly experienced in their research, when asked what the meaning of their lives might be, people may be embarrassed, answer with a blank expression on their faces, or ask what is meant by 'meaning'. This ambiguity is clearly apparent in the philosophical and social science literature. Some authors define life meaning mystically as pertaining to one's relationship with God, or with one's soul, or both; others relate it to creativity and the benefit this has to other people. At the same time, there is no consensus regarding whether the meaning in life is subjective (experiential) or objective (has observable characteristics beyond individual experiences), or both.

General propositions

McNamee (2007) defines life meaning concisely as 'a sense that a person has that life is worth living' (p. 1 of 15). Many other scholars consider meaning to be a much more complex phenomenon which emerges out of an individual's total experience through 'the interaction of subjects, objects, elements or situations' (Peterson, 2000, p. 1 of 24). This experience has a narrative: it consists of preceding actions (either on the part of the person who is experiencing or other people or environmental elements around the individual), and is followed by consequences. In this sense, meaning is existential since it comes out of choices, actions, and consequences; it is phenomenological, since it relies on the individual interpretation of events; and according to Frankl (1969), it depends on concrete actions geared towards fulfilling a specific mission in life, making it experiential.

As the existential aspect of meaning 'relies on definitions of truth manifested in action and then tested by the consequences of such action,' (Peterson, 2000, p. 1 of 24) it is also motivational in the sense that it relates to practical needs. The search for food, shelter, warmth, and security is existentially meaningful since it pertains to a person's need to construct and destroy things, rejuvenate the being, and inhabit the world; growing food, burning fuel, and building dwellings as part of the strategy for survival. This relationship between survival (an existential need) and meaning is reflected even in childhood play. Winnicott (1971) suggested that play (as a concrete action) is naturally connected to reality in the sense that it fulfills a natural need arising from the process of human development. The playful interaction between a child and her mother engenders a process of primary socialization. The child develops a bond with the mother and comes to realize that she is not alone in the world. The child begins to appreciate boundaries to her existence. Developing an awareness of the environment enables the child to develop increasingly subtle ways of communicating with her mother. A key stage of this development is the ability to symbolize the continuity of the mother's presence in order for the child to feel secure. When the mother is temporarily absent the child has to understand that she will return to nurture her and that her continued existence is not in jeopardy. This recognition makes further exploration of the environment possible enhancing the possibility of encountering more meaningful experiences. Thus the child's sense of meaning is derived from the assurance of continued existential survival.

Peterson (2000) and Frankl (1992) suggested that meaningfulness is associated existentially with **goal setting, or with worthwhile goals towards which to aspire**. Goal setting is based on knowledge of the objective world and its challenges, and the evaluation of previous actions to achieve articulated goals geared towards meeting them. One of the occupational therapy approaches to goal setting developed by du Toit (2009) consisted of a stepped understanding of recovery. Recovery was conceptualized to progress from a positive 'tone' (du Toit, 2009, p. 23) indicating the undeveloped potential for action, through to stages of increasing participation. In her work, Du Toit (who was partly informed by Frankl's ideas) was concerned with the idea of 'creative ability' (2009, p. 22) and a spiralling capacity and potential which increased with experience and the ability to anticipate the pleasure that could result from taking up opportunities for engagement. A key component of this idea was the relationship between volition, motivated by setting goals which were just within the capacity of the recovering individual, and performance. The goals would not be motivational if they could not be realised. Ikiugu (2005) and Ikiugu and Rosso (2005) describe such goals as occupational life trajectory attractors because they provide meaning to, and therefore organize, patterns of performance as individuals interact with and act within the environment. For example, if a person wants to become a doctor then it is probable that he or she will prefer to engage in the kinds of actions that are consistent with the achievement of this goal, such as studying, volunteering in appropriate tasks, looking for opportunities at careers fairs to find out details about suitable university courses, etc. (Ikiugu, 2005).

Ikiugu (2005), and Ikiugu and Rosso (2005) suggest that this occupational pattern forms a trajectory for an individual's life or what du Toit (2009) might refer to as a person's developing creative ability over time. This suggests that meaning can be defined as a phenomenon that arises out of the creativity in a person's activities over a given period in his or her life. For example, a span of time during which a person may be seeking voluntary work and exploring different university courses could later be understood by the person as 'the time when I was deciding to become a doctor'. Thus, action, creativity, and meaning may be perceived to be intertwined. Frankl (1992) argued that an ultimate embodiment of meaning would be the act of doing something as an expression of an individual's love or need for another person or a thing. Ideally, the experience of successful doing enables a person to visualize goals and to plan actions towards complex outcomes. Actions which may be most meaningful may fulfill a need to express love for another person or a concept – perhaps a principle or an institution. Ultimately a combination of actions may constitute an expression of hope for a future that structures one's life trajectory (Ikiugu, 2005; Ikiugu & Rosso, 2005), and the vision of this future may be best articulated in a worthwhile mission in life (Frankl, 1997; Krasko, 1997, see also Ikiugu, 2011, 2008, 2007, 2004a, 2004b, 2004c). More discussion of this notion can be found in chapter 6.

This does not suggest that people have to be anxious about whether or not their actions always contribute optimally towards worthwhile life goals. Most everyday human actions are not connected to the fulfillment of ideals or to the creation of a desired legacy. In a complex world it is difficult to make predictions about the outcomes of performance. Sometimes, as Kazez (2007) suggests, the best we can hope for as we engage in our daily tasks in life is to be just 'good enough'. She points out that 'our lives would seem far less interesting if it were really possible to approach them with an instruction manual' (pp. 157-158). This is the case even in important roles such as that of being parents, who, Winnicott (1971) thought, had to be just 'good enough'. Part of human socialization involves realizing that we are probably capable of determining what actions to take to achieve important goals in life, without becoming anxious or obsessive about it.

The literature reviewed for this chapter suggests that meaning is composed of more than worthwhile goals or a mission in life. It also has a function of giving one an experience of coherence and continuity, order, inner harmony, value, and the ability to make choices and to act (Dwyer, Nordenfelt, & Ternestdt, 2008; Fleer, Hoekstra, Sleijfer et al., 2006; Jim & Andersen, 2007; Thompson,

2007). The perception of coherence as a source of meaning includes being aware of reminiscence, through which people use their past experiences to shape a desired future. People often find value in relating the past to their children and grandchildren, thus satisfying the curiosity of younger generations about earlier times (Vincent, 1981). The activity of describing the past contributes to the future coherence of society by sustaining cultural and spiritual knowledge.

Chodorow (1989, 1978) suggests that the shape and form given to this transmission of cultural and spiritual values may offer differing forms of continuity among the genders – men are encouraged as boys to be independent, while women as girls are encouraged to be interdependent. These differences are reflected in the continuous and unbroken phylogenetic relationships between mothers and their daughters, whereas those between fathers and sons are often disrupted. These different patterns of coherence result in gendered approaches to making sense of the world. Individual affirmation is experienced through interdependence in the case of women and through independence by conquest and the exercise of power over others in the case of men. The male oriented social structure of dominance has been a result of valuing of independence and conquest rather than interdependence, which is a priority for women (Irigaray, 1993). The neutral individual depicted in philosophy or in the desexualized language of non-sexism thus still remains an expression of male identity in a society in which women's way of being in the world is not fully acknowledged.

Occupational therapists and occupational scientists are members of a professional and academic community composed predominantly of women. For the profession of occupational therapy to recognize a critical notion of meaning, the influence of its strongly gendered constituency has to be addressed. As Frank (1992) noted in her exploration of the feminist history of occupational therapy, while women have felt empowered in the profession, they have also maintained a narrow cultural base represented by white middle class women's perspective, a group whose expression of meaning may reflect a certain degree of class privilege. The profession has had to struggle for its objectives and resources in the male ordered hegemonies of health care (Pollard & Walsh, 2000). However, in order to survive it has to engage with clients in a diverse society which presents a wider range of cultural meanings and understandings of occupation (Sakellariou & Pollard, 2008). While occupational therapy practice is supposed to focus on clients' needs, its feminine cultural perspective may not reflect the lived experiences of males with disabilities (Block et al, 2012; Sakellariou & Pollard, 2012), whose needs (in the areas of productivity, self-care, social participation, intimacy, etc.) are different from those of female clients. Occupational therapists have to attract and support the development of a much wider professional membership, and a great variety of tools and approaches to work equally and holistically with all clients. As a source of underpinning theory and evidence for occupation, occupational science has a similar task of investigating the diverse phenomena of meaning in doing.

According to Peterson (2000), there are three levels of meaning:

1. meaning of the determined world which arises out of the human tendency to simplify reality so that it can be comprehended;
2. meaning related to novelty, which comes out of fulfillment of human curiosity and need to explore; and
3. meaning arising out of the interaction between determined world and satisfaction of curiosity and need to explore, which is one of the factors involved in comprehending determined world to enhance human survival.

Meaningfulness as a function of one's relationship with God, soul, or both

In Diane's account at the beginning of the book, she placed a great deal of importance on religious interpretations of life meaning. As mentioned earlier, most human cultures maintain a significant concern with spiritual activities carried out by individuals. Many people perceive meaning to be connected to a relationship with a higher power such as God [also referred to as 'God-centered meaning'] or to one's soul [also referred to as 'soul-centered meaning'] (Metz, 2007). The God-centered view is based on the notion that meaning results from fulfilling God's purpose or working within God's plan for the universe. Gordon (1983) argued that God endows us with meaning in the same way that artists breathe meaning into their creations. Indeed adherents of most religions suggest that their gods were directly involved in the creation of the world. It follows that for people holding such beliefs, God is necessary for meaning because in their perception, individual human lives are finite and therefore cannot be meaningful by themselves (Nozick, 1989, 1981).

In most Western traditions, finiteness (or mortality) denotes imperfection, a state which lacks meaning, and therefore, in many religious systems doing good deeds is considered a public responsibility, a way of striving for the perfection of immortality in heaven. God's perfection and the extended notion of this perfection to heaven are infinite sources of meaning to humans' finite lives. Christians often presume that by living well they can attain perfection in an afterlife through admission into heaven, although they cannot assume perfection in their finite lives. Thus there is a distinction between what is cosmically meaningful because it is infinite and what is fleetingly meaningful because it is finite.

In some Judeo Christian and Islamic perspectives, perfection is a state that is beyond human comprehension; there can be no attribution of human values to God, since God is beyond human understanding (Jones, 1984). In Buddhism, nirvana is a state of perfection through enlightenment, i.e. a state of understanding that should eventually lead to loss of separate individuality and spiritual merging with a primordial consciousness. In this system of thought, perfection occurs by relinquishing aspects of the self in order to attain enlightenment by merging with the ultimate cosmic consciousness (Suzuki, 1969; Trungpa, 1973)

In many religions, human lives are understood to be equally meaningful because they derive their meaning from God or a primordial consciousness. Never the less, as Dorling (2011, p. 2) illustrates, the reality is that religious teaching has little impact on people's sensibilities about 'elitism, exclusion, prejudice, greed and despair', the 'five beliefs', which produce victims who can be categorized as 'the delinquents, the debarred, the discarded, the debtors and the depressed'. Religions have often taught that these conditions are the results of sin, or constitute a temporary period of suffering. While this teaching may have the function of encouraging resiliency through hope, it may also serve to sustain the status quo and preserve order in society by encouraging people to accept and bear suffering without complaining, as a necessary condition of their lot. Consequently the beliefs of the powerful have often been endorsed by religion while social criticism and negotiation by the disenfranchised for better conditions have been constrained by religious teachings (King, 2000; Rowland, 1988). Though at times a strong sense of spirituality has been a force in support of challenge to the status quo, religious ideas have instead for the most part acted as a brake to progressive social change and instead become a force for conservatism (Jones, 1984; King, 2000; Luthuli, 1963; Mandela, 1994; Rowland 1988; Torres, 1973). In some societies, as McFarland and Matthews (2005) found in their study, the characteristic of holding religious values appeared to be associated with less regard for human rights. The rights of lesbian, gay, bisexual, and transgender individuals, the ordination of women, and the recognition of past abuses in religious institutions are significant issues with which elements of the established churches have had to reconcile themselves during the early part of the 21st century.

It is also noteworthy that various religious systems hold different beliefs and values which affect the life meanings which may be associated with them. For example, Buddhism is a practice or belief system that might outwardly be described as a religion, but most Buddhists may be unconcerned with such definitions which would stand in the way of seeking truth by generating divisions between people. Because of this principle of tolerance, it follows that Buddhists may be able to live meaningful lives side by side with people holding a diversity of beliefs. It might be desirable for religions to be similarly flexible in their outlook towards others with the realization that there is a plurality of possibilities by which life meaning and purpose can be experienced, and one view, including a religious one, does not monopolize the notion of meaning in life. However, many of the Buddhist scriptures identify episodes of violence arising from disputes between different followers, and war and violence persists where Buddhism dominates amongst other religious identities in societies such as Sri Lanka. The cause of these conflicts, according to Buddhist belief, is usually human sensual desires and material greed, but the reality may involve many factors including nationalism and cultural conflict (Degalle, 2006). In other words, whatever spiritual aspirations people may have, their everyday lives are grounded in material issues which may weigh down on their ideals. If we strive to do, be, become, and belong through meaningful occupational engagement (Wilcock, 2006), then some of the conditions that make human occupations meaningful and purposeful may include negative as well as positive possibilities of what we can become; unwelcome experiences may give rise to good outcomes, and vice versa. In the end, for humanity to have a chance of living meaningful lives, there must be a conceptualization of meaning that does not deny the finite nature and imperfection of human life (Metz, 2007; Quinn, 2000).

Finally, critics of the necessity of God or a higher power for establishment of a meaningful life contest the idea that imperfect beings can have a relationship with an infinite presence. They claim that such an idea is simply absurd, since finite humans cannot understand an infinite being. As understanding is a prerequisite for a relationship, and as human beings cannot really understand an infinite god, there is no way for humans to derive meaningfulness from a relationship with such a god. If on the other hand we can relate to that presence, then god cannot be perfect because it is a product of human conceptualization. If a god is beyond human understanding then it cannot be perceived as such. This argument, which Berger (1973, p. 106) terms 'methodological atheism', stems from the idea that all concepts of god are human projections. Viewed this way, it is impossible to say that God existed before humans, since humans have only become aware of God by learning religious practices from each other.

Of course, humans can understand something as complex as an infinite universe even if it is unlikely that they will understand everything about it. In Adams' (1979) *The Hitchhiker's Guide to the Galaxy* (p. 135), he describes a futuristic computer ('Deep Thought'), whose purpose is to find the answer to the ultimate question of Life; the secret of the Universe and Everything in it. The answer to the question turns out to be 'forty two'. According to Adams, the answer could not be understood by humans because they 'didn't know what the question is [...] and once you do know what the question is, you'll know what it means' (p. 136). Never the less, humans could apprehend the meaning of 'forty two' even though they did not understand how the computer obtained the answer. Thus, it is not necessary to understand everything in order to develop a conception of meaning. Humans recognize each other and various capacities and attributes shared with others even though they still do not understand everything about their fellow beings and are unlikely to fully understand themselves. Occupational therapists necessarily have to confront this issue if they are to develop a holistic perspective of the human being, which is a cornerstone of the new professional paradigm (American Occupational Therapy Association, 2014; Kielhofner, 2009). Holistic thinking suggests taking into account the immense complexity of the human being, of almost infinite proportions.

The problem of the finite contemplating the infinite is not one of attempting to understand something without boundaries, but of understanding that something has the capacity to exist without limits. For example, according to scientists, the universe is in an expanding state (Hawking, 1994, 1988). Since it is expanding, it makes logical sense that at one time it was extremely small, and therefore we can assume that it had a beginning, which scientists have postulated to be the big bang. This gives rise to the question, what happened before the big bang? If there had been a previous expansion and contraction prior to this event, does the universe have a cyclical nature, in that it must at some point contract leading to another big bang, then expand, then contract again, and infinitum? This is an example of a conceptualization of co-existence of the infinite and finite realities. In the cosmic sense, infinity as expressed in the cyclical expansion and contraction of the universe over vast time periods can be seen as necessary for a finite life. If this theory is correct, there is a balance between finiteness and infinity, since each episode between big bangs is finite, while the process of expansion and contraction as a whole is infinite. The existence of everything depends on this infinite pulsation.

This leads us to the assertion that whether or not they accept the existence of a God, human beings have to come to terms with their mortality and the continuation of the world and the wider universe around them for eternity. Many people deal with their mortality by taking a specific series of actions that make their lives sensible. Some establish legacies for future generations by sharing memories and life narratives. In this way people are able to see the meaning of their own finite existence in relation to the continuous life of the universe. In this sense, the ritual of mourning, arranging funerals and dealing with the personal effects and affairs of someone who has died can be seen as an affirmation of the continuation of existence for those who are still living (Pollard, 2006).

The soul-centered view of meaningfulness on the other hand is based on the idea that a soul is an eternal substance within us (not limited like our material bodies), and therefore it is immortal and perfect (Metz, 2007). Therefore, individual lives can only have meaning by people having the ability to do things that express the soul, since only the soul has immortality and permanence. The objection to this perspective again arises from the fact that there is no evidence of the existence of a soul, let alone the question of whether having a soul necessarily denotes immortality or lack thereof.

Often the soul is thought to be an expression of the human spirit, but such metaphysical concepts, like gods, derive from human mythologies. These mythologies are used not only to explain the universe but also to control social behaviors and activities which religious authorities perceive as threats to social stability. Thus, by explaining the order of the physical universe they establish a basis for human conduct in the social realm. What is important to bear in mind is that the conceptualization of the nature of the cosmos determines (but since it is a mythological conceptualization it is also determined by) how people shall live.

However, mythologies are analogous to what has evolved into scientific explanation. The two systems aim at the same goal, which is to make the universe comprehensible to human beings. While mythology is a metaphorical way of visualizing the universe, science attempts to reveal the literal explanatory logic behind its mechanism. Of course adherents of religion sometimes assert that their views of the universe are literal rather than metaphorical, and scientists sometimes come to terms with their discoveries by understanding them in terms of religious metaphor. That is why many scientists believe in the existence of God (for example both Einstein and Newton were firm believers in the existence of God as the intelligent architect who established the laws governing the universe). Nevertheless, critics argue that neither an infinite soul nor any metaphysical thing exerting an infinite effect on the world is necessary for a meaningful life (Schmidtz, 2001).

Objective versus subjective views

With such a diverse range of arguments, it is not surprising that some scholars claim that meaning is idiosyncratic (Metz, 2007). In other words, meaning derives from subjective experiences which are unique to every individual, and thus, if anyone believes that something is meaningful, then it is. Therefore, meaning is primarily a result of the achievement of goals that people individually set for themselves. However, meaning is also related to the interpretation of objective phenomena, things which remain relatively constant, such as the landscape or the seasons, and the relative permanence of some social institutions. Metz (2007, p. 11 of 21) suggested that 'subjectivism about meaning has lost dominance over the past thirty years'. This is probably because of increased secularization of western populations and the growing power of science combined with the development of technology and of the financial structures in a global society. For example, people expect product reliability. They expect certainty, and many of the products they use are supported by an increasingly complex technology. An expectation of perfection does not so much reside in the almighty, but has become humanized in the mobile phone, the bank service, better evidence, the digitalization of information, and the reduction of anticipated risk in life.

On the other hand, the objective view is based on the proposition that 'there are certain inherently worthwhile or finally valuable conditions that confer meaning for anyone, not merely because they are wanted, chosen, or believed to be meaningful, nor because they somehow are grounded in God' (Metz, 2007, p. 12 of 21). In other words, objectivists submit that there are external criteria for meaning on which everyone can agree. Once those criteria are met in a person's life, it can be assumed that the individual's life is meaningful. Those who define meaning in this way tend to equate it with moral and creative actions that can be judged objectively as worthwhile: 'the activities that give meaning to one's life will give one reasons for acting that are, to some extent, independent of self-interest – reasons derived from the worth of the activities themselves' (Paul, Miller, & Paul, 1997, p. xii). This understanding of meaning still has inherent difficulties. One group of people may decide that promoting a particular set of beliefs is a worthwhile moral and creative action, while another may object on different moral grounds which they hold to be significant. Although a society or a group agrees on criteria for meaning, it does not follow that their opinion represents the true reality of the phenomenon. For many years it was supposed that the earth was the centre of the universe, that it was flat, and that the sun revolved around it. Everyone at the time thought that this was objective truth. Now it is understood, on the basis of irrefutable evidence, that the earth's position in the universe is very different. It is dawning on the earthlings that the importance of the earth is only to the people living on it. The wider significance of the planet and the life on it may be very small given the infinity of space. Thus, history is full of surprises which have changed common understandings of reality.

This issue of objective versus subjective definition of meaning takes us back to the argument about the role of finiteness versus infinity in meaning-making. For example, you want to know that your computer works and is reliable. However, you may not understand very much about how it works and probably never will. All you need to know is how to use the computer. But there are many computers on the market with similar characteristics. One of the subjective judgments (subjective because you accept the information given to you by the technical experts on faith) you have to make is to buy a particular model based on the apparently objective criteria (such as memory size, processing speed, type of interphase, number of apps, available technological assistance, etc.) presented to you by the supplier. You do not buy the computer purely on the basis of explicit objective criteria that you fully understand such as colour (although such criteria may be part of the equation in your decision-making). You don't really understand much of the information the tech gives you about the computer, except that it sounds pretty good and the tech sounds and looks competent to you. You do not actually test much of the computer capabilities yourself before you buy it, but rather you buy it on the basis of a subjective judgment of the extent to which you can trust the information given to you by the techs.

According to Adams (1979), this is the same kind of judgment on which understanding of the Universe and everything in it is based. The idea that forty two may be the answer to the question 'what is the meaning of life' may be as good as any other, and viewed in this sense, the difference between subject and object is illusory: people are often persuaded that many things are objective. Indeed, many things may actually be objective to the best of the knowledge of the people developing the information about them, but that information is still understood, disseminated and used by individuals based on choices which are based on subjective judgment. Subjective choices are for example governing how this book is being written. We have been persuaded to write it in order to deal with professional and scientific questions which may be objective. However, our interest and motivation is subjective, just as the reader is perhaps motivated by subjective reasons to read this textbook.

Many scholars take the middle ground, and we (speaking of ourselves subjectively) tend to agree with this position. They see the judgement of meaningful actions as having both objective and subjective components. An action may be reckoned to be meaningful in the consensus of wider society, but some individuals may not recognize it as meaningful to them. There may often be common assumptions about shared interests from which some people are excluded. For example, in many Western societies it is assumed that most people can read, but there are people who experience difficulties with reading, and therefore cannot share in the enjoyment of books or magazines and the meanings these activities may have for people in general. Books and magazines and the activity of reading may have no meaning for these people, despite the rich meaning they have for others.

Nihilists and Taoists dispute the idea that life has any meaning at all (Nagel, 1986) other than as a flicker in the temporal scale of the universe, and therefore is virtually un-important. For them, pre-occupation with the search for meaning is a reflection of human arrogance, a lack of perspective, and is utterly futile. Instead, Taoists might argue, everything is a part of the void, it is both something and nothing, and rather than searching for meaning, we should accept experience as it is for the pleasure of experience.

A working definition of meaningfulness

There are some apparently contradictory perspectives in this discussion. A Taoist view of meaning contains meaninglessness, not as indifference to reality, but as acceptance of it. A Western perspective might generally be that: 'A meaningful life…is a life of active engagement in projects of worth, which might involve such things as moral or intellectual accomplishments, relationships with family and friends, or artistic/creative enterprises' (Paul et al., 1997, p. xii). Meaning can also be defined as an experience of coherence, as well as a sense of creativity and control over the span of one's life (Carlson, Clark, & Young, 1998). Dwyer, Nordenfelt, and Ternestedt (2008, p. 98) offer a particularly relevant definition of the construct thus: 'Meaning is understood here in general sense of one's self and one's life having a value, within a focus on everyday life.' Human society is based on co-operation and participation, which suggests a perception of and need for shared values. The core theme of this book is that individuals need to live meaningfully through what they do in the pursuit of daily occupations, and suggests a common sense approach to a working definition of meaningfulness, based in tacit knowledge and derived from experience.

As De Certeau (1988) found in his exploration of the practice of everyday life, things which are close at hand are meaningful because they are immediately useful. The way in which people associate with others in the community in which they live is through a common knowledge of where to get a decent cut of meat, or a meeting at their preferred café which they get to through a short cut through the streets which they know of, and at which they might discuss how to get a new job, or where they can have their car fixed. These are examples of how people get by in work or life in general. The commonsense understanding of meaningfulness lies in this sense of connectedness with other people and with one's context, and is realized through a mosaic of the mundane.

The paradox of the objective/subjective definition of meaning is apparent in the key skill of establishing rapport with clients in the client centered approach to therapy. The therapist has to listen carefully to the client. Even where the client has difficulty in engaging, the therapist has to provide an opportunity for him/her to communicate (du Toit, 2009). Despite the expertise of the therapist, the will to act rests with the client. The client's lived experience qualifies him/her to challenge the therapist's knowledge, however objective that knowledge might be in the perspective of the therapist (Sinclair, 2007). To appreciate and come to terms with the kind of knowledge such lived experience may reveal, therapists may have to prepare, just as they would when they study in order to expand their clinical and theoretical knowledge, by developing their awareness of and accepting other perspectives of meaningfulness. This entails being aware of the subjectivities which have been absorbed through the process of becoming a therapist, or the culture and society in which one grew up. These subjective contexts provide individuals with ideological definitions of meaning that exclude recognition of the experiences of other people. For example, even in occupational therapy education, Beagan (2007) found that working class occupational therapy students tended not to discuss personal experiences in class because the dominant middle class milieu of the university made them feel insignificant. They thought that what they said would simply not be heard, an indication that they were made to feel that their lives were not as meaningful as those of their more privileged classmates.

As healthcare workers, occupational therapists often deal with problems that arise from social and economic disparities and their consequences on health. The knowledge that professionals use is often learned as a set of technical interventions. These are often presented as specialized forms of knowledge, applied in clinical settings; whereas the conditions being treated are experienced quite differently by the people who are being treated (Frank, 1995; Mattingly, 1998). The experiences of anxiety, discomfort, pain, disability, the disruption of life narratives, and the social narratives which clients have, can be explained to but not always shared experientially with the therapist. The life trajectory of the therapist may often be different from that of the client in many respects, and each may experience subjective differences in the definition of meaning and what is meaningful.

In this chapter we have very broadly discussed various perspectives of meaningfulness. Our concern remains to explore how daily occupational life may be used to enhance meaning in peoples' lives. One of the things that we want to emphasize though, because there often is a misunderstanding, is that meaning should not be confused with happiness. As Belliotti (2001, p. 129) stated: 'Meaningful lives...are not necessarily happy lives'. Frankl (1992) certainly understood this because he experienced persecution and many losses but came to recognize that painful events may be meaningful. Many people who choose to relate their experiences in writing describe periods of pain and struggle. African National Congress leaders Alfred Luthuli (1963) and Nelson Mandela (1994) and civil rights leader Martin Luther King, Jr. (2000) are examples. Like many of the worker writers whose lives are explored in the next chapter, the meaningfulness they appear to have experienced did not preclude moments of unbearable pain and unhappiness.

Thus, it is difficult to know for sure how happy individuals who have lived meaningful lives were. Readers can only project their experiences empathically onto them in the form of thinking 'I would be happy, or unhappy, if I was in their circumstances'. Despite the difficulties they endured, including imprisonment, physical violence, loss of loved ones and friends, and threats to their lives, none of the people listed in the above examples lived their entire lives in distress. King (2000) certainly understood himself to have a destiny to fulfill and seemed to have faced the possibility of assassination with equanimity. What we want to underscore, as stated earlier, is that a meaningful life is not necessarily a happy one, since meaning and happiness are not inextricably linked, although, '... happy lives, at least those that are not artificially induced, are invariably meaningful' (Belliotti, 2001, p. 129). In other words, meaningfulness does not equate with happiness, but happiness always subsumes meaningfulness.

Note

1 There are those who argue that bad as the working conditions were in factories, such conditions were still better for factory workers than for those in rural areas. Drucker (1993) for example argued that even though it was true that the conditions in factories during the industrial revolution period were indeed abysmal, factory workers often enjoyed a higher standard of living and experienced a higher life expectancy than their rural counterparts.

Applying the ideas discussed in Chapter 1

Think of a client with whom you are working right now. Bearing the issues of concern for this client in mind, think about the following:

- Based on the discussion in chapter 1, what is your understanding of the construct 'meaning in life'?
- Based on that personal understanding of what meaning in life entails, and your understanding of the issues of priority for your client, what do you think is the status of your client's meaning in life (or lack there-of)?

A quick appraisal of your client's sense of meaning in life

Ask your client to rate himself on how meaningful he perceives his life to be at the moment using the rating scale in the following assessment.

Caution: The indicators of meaning in life in the self-assessment below are based on propositions in the reviewed literature. Please explain to the client that the purpose of the self-assessment is to enable the client to identify areas of her internal experience of life in which she could increase satisfaction. This has nothing to do with whether or not her life is meaningful in any objective sense, as an internal experience is not something that can be measured externally by observers. The client may even be able to think of other indicators of meaning in her life that are not listed here. If she does so encourage her to list them in the 'Other Indicators of Meaning in your Life' category and rate herself on them accordingly.

Ensure that the client understands that a low score in this self-assessment does not mean that his life is meaningless or worthless, but it merely means that perhaps in the client's mind, he could optimize meaning for increased satisfaction with his life. Irrespective of what we feel about how our lives are going, it would be wise to remember that if we ask those close to us, they will probably tell us that our lives are immeasurably important to them irrespective of our accomplishments and failures. Ultimately, an individual is the best judge of personal circumstances and in the end it is the individual's opinions and feelings about life that matter.

Fig 1.1: Assessment of perceived meaning in life

ASSESSMENT OF PERCEPTION OF MEANING IN LIFE

Indicator of Meaning in Life	**Perception of How often it is True in an Individual's Life**				
	Always True	**Often True**	**Neither True nor False**	**Rarely True**	**Never True**
1. I feel positive emotions	[ ]	[ ]	[ ]	[ ]	[ ]
2. I experience my life as having a purpose	[ ]	[ ]	[ ]	[ ]	[ ]
3. I have a meaningful philosophy that guides my life	[ ]	[ ]	[ ]	[ ]	[ ]
4. I have worthwhile goals to which I aspire in my life	[ ]	[ ]	[ ]	[ ]	[ ]
5. I am in control of my life	[ ]	[ ]	[ ]	[ ]	[ ]
6. I find ways of solving problems that come up in my life	[ ]	[ ]	[ ]	[ ]	[ ]
7. I pursue my life goals with enthusiasm and energy	[ ]	[ ]	[ ]	[ ]	[ ]
8. I am hopeful that my future will be good	[ ]	[ ]	[ ]	[ ]	[ ]
9. My work is a positive part of who I am	[ ]	[ ]	[ ]	[ ]	[ ]
10. My work utilizes my abilities optimally	[ ]	[ ]	[ ]	[ ]	[ ]
11. My work makes me feel that I am a valued contributing member of society	[ ]	[ ]	[ ]	[ ]	[ ]
12. I participate in activities that transcend my pursuit of personal pleasure	[ ]	[ ]	[ ]	[ ]	[ ]
13. I feel connected to my community	[ ]	[ ]	[ ]	[ ]	[ ]
14. The things I do in my work and other activities contribute to something bigger than myself	[ ]	[ ]	[ ]	[ ]	[ ]
15. I do things that make me feel happy and fulfilled	[ ]	[ ]	[ ]	[ ]	[ ]
16. I feel capable	[ ]	[ ]	[ ]	[ ]	[ ]
17. I feel culturally connected	[ ]	[ ]	[ ]	[ ]	[ ]

Other Indicators of Meaning in your Life (Please, List)	**Perception of How True it is in an Individual's Life**				
	Always True	**Often True**	**Neither True nor False**	**Rarely True**	**Never True**
1.	[ ]	[ ]	[ ]	[ ]	[ ]
2.	[ ]	[ ]	[ ]	[ ]	[ ]
3.	[ ]	[ ]	[ ]	[ ]	[ ]
4.	[ ]	[ ]	[ ]	[ ]	[ ]
5.	[ ]	[ ]	[ ]	[ ]	[ ]
6.	[ ]	[ ]	[ ]	[ ]	[ ]
7.	[ ]	[ ]	[ ]	[ ]	[ ]
Total Perception of Meaning Score (add all the ratings above to obtain your client's total score)					[ ]

Scoring Codes for the Meaningfulness Scale:

Never True = 1

Rarely True = 2

Neither True nor False = 3

Often True = 4

Always True = 5

Note: The items in the scale were derived from extensive literature review. In particular, the following sources were used: Feldman and Snyder (2005), Iwasaki (2007), Mascaro and Rosen (2005), and Michaelson (2007)

Chapter 2 Meaningfulness as an experienced phenomenon: Lessons from worker-writer autobiographies

Learning objectives

After reading this chapter which is based on the findings in the study by Ikiugu et al. (2012), the reader will understand how:

1. The English Worker-Writers whose autobiographies were analysed experienced themselves as meaning-makers in their lives
2. The experiences of the English Worker-Writers can be used to help people understand how their daily occupations contribute to meaning-making in their lives

Contents of this chapter

- What makes occupations meaningful?
- People use occupations to construct/discover meaning in their lives by using them to:
    - Connect to something bigger than themselves
    - Create a sense of fulfilment through exploration and creativity
    - Connect to other people
    - Have a sense of social responsibility
    - Experience a sense of efficacy/competence, and independence
    - Experience a sense of dignity
    - Experience affirmation of their identity as individuals
    - Make personal life stories
    - Create experiences that are relevant to their developmental stage
    - Demonstrate ability to negotiate change and to adapt
    - Experience a sense of Intimacy
    - Transition through life
    - Create a place for themselves in the cultural and temporal context

Introduction

In the last chapter we explored Frankl's notion that people have come to see their lives as empty and lacking in meaning and purpose, with a corresponding decline in a sense of well-being. Elaborating on Frankl's proposition, Royce (1964, p. 76) went so far as to propose that: 'about all that remains of humanity is an outer shell, for the 'inner man' is on his last legs. And the 20th century neurosis is the neurosis of purposelessness, meaninglessness, value-lessness, hollowness, or emptiness'. We concluded that meaningfulness may not always be associated with happiness (and perhaps not even wellbeing), but happiness was connected with meaningfulness. In his Ruth Zemke lecture in occupational science Rowles (2008) stated that: 'The ultimate focus of each human life is a search for meaning' (p. 127). He went on to emphasize that: 'once the essentials of survival have been met, a primary focus of life is the discovery of meaning' (p. 128). In this book, we argue that occupational therapists and occupational scientists have the skills to help people meet this desire to discover meaning in their lives. The profession has developed a specialized knowledge that can be used to assist people in making choices and strategizing about how to adequately perform daily occupations that maximize meaning in their lives.

Of course helping people experience their lives as meaningful is a relevant domain of practice for many other professionals including psychologists, philosophers, and psychological counsellors among others. However, occupational therapists and occupational scientists are particularly suited to understand the role of daily occupations in this endeavour. The current belief among occupational therapy and occupational science scholars is that meaningful occupation is associated with a sense of well-being among human beings (Christiansen, 2000, 1999; Matuska & Christiansen, 2008; Tatzer, van Nes, & Jonsson, 2011), and 'Meaningfulness' is one of the core constructs in the new occupational therapy paradigm (American Occupational Therapy Association [AOTA], 2014; Canadian Association of Occupational Therapists [CAOT], 2002; Kielhofner, 2009).

Since the 1990s, many occupational therapy and occupational science scholars have investigated the relationship between daily occupations and meaning in life. Schemm and Gitlin (1993) noted that using meaningful activity as a medium for therapeutic interventions created a sense of fulfilment and investment in therapy among occupational therapy clients. However, they acknowledged that identifying meaningful occupations for use in therapy is a complex process. Hasselkus (2002) investigated how meaningful daily occupations provided the medium through which life flowed for individuals living in long term care facilities. Hammell (2004) stated that depression, which is prevalent in the Western Societies in spite of material affluence, can be averted if people are able to find meaning in every-day activities. Matuska and Christiansen (2008) explored the relationship between occupation and life balance. They proposed that the creation of meaning and the ability to identify aspects of life as meaningful was an essential component of a positive and healthy life balance.

Christiansen (1999) proposed that life stories derived from an understanding of what people do in contexts was the occupational basis for development of personal identities. Tatzer, van Nes, and Jonsson (2011) used life stories to demonstrate how a small group of women maintained their occupational identities over their lifetimes, one aspect of which was their sense of struggle. Earlier Lentin (2002) had explored how the concept of survival was significant in creating a life despite traumatic experiences, and had suggested that the experience of trauma may be widespread in human society.

Lentin (2002) made a claim that 'meaningfulness' is a core professional construct, but understanding it in occupational therapy and occupational science terms is quite different from applying it in practice. Over the same period in which these studies relating occupation and meaning have been conducted, criticism has come from both within (Townsend 1998; Townsend, Langille, & Ripley, 2003) and outside occupational therapy, challenging the profession's claim that it is occupation-centered (based on use of meaningful occupations as therapeutic media) and client-centered (Abberley, 1995). Many occupational therapists have noted that it is difficult to always use meaningful occupations as therapeutic media within a biomedical framework of practice (Wilding & Whiteford, 2007), which is increasingly constrained by budgetary and productivity concerns. Occupational therapists, like many other health care professionals and clients

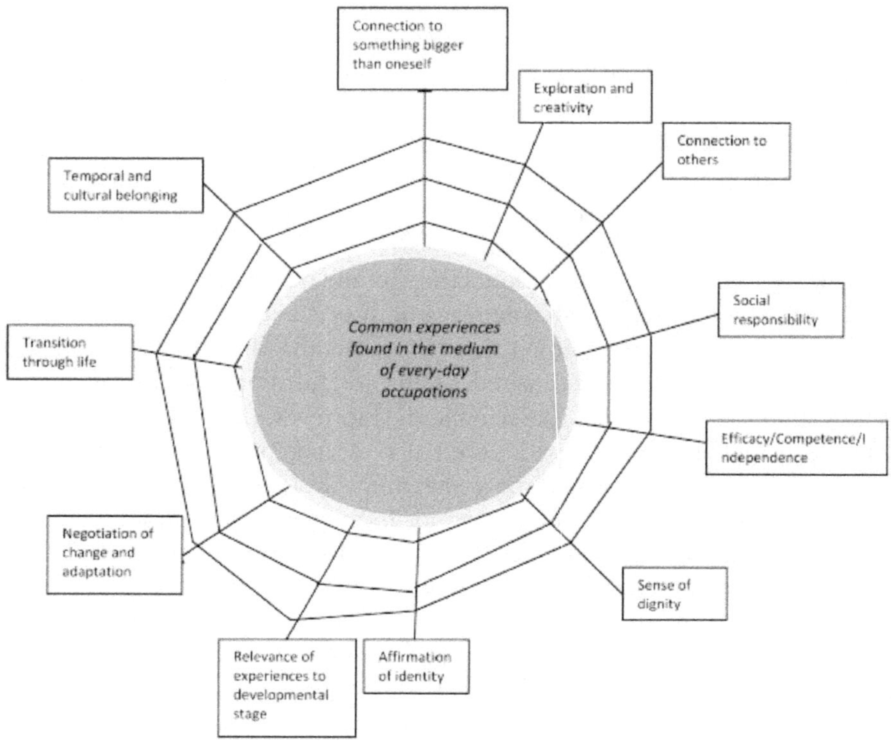

Common experiences found in every-day occupations are depicted as the medium through which meaning in life emerges. Through engagement in daily occupations and subsequent experiences in occupational participation, the individual constructs meaning in his/her life by: connecting to something bigger than him/herself; engaging in self-exploration and creativity; connecting to other people; having a sense of social responsibility; having a sense of efficacy, competence, and independence; having a sense of dignity; affirming his/her unique identity; perceiving the experiences as relevant to his/her developmental stage; negotiating change and adapting; transitioning through life; and having a sense of temporal and cultural belonging.

Figure 2-1. Web of meaning through daily occupational performance.

themselves, are concerned with what Rowles (2008) calls 'essentials of survival', which include paying the bills and staying in work rather than adhering to the core values such as occupation-based and client-centered practice (Hammell, 2010, 2008, 2007; Rebiero-Gruhl, 2009). The pressures generated by the need to reconcile core professional philosophy with economic survival pose a concern as to whether occupational therapy can remain true to its tenets that justify its existence in the first place, and still continue to remain viable.

To be able to practice in a way that is consistent with the professional value of meaningfulness occupational therapists need to clearly and comprehensively define what makes occupations meaningful. Without this clarity it is difficult for them to play their proper role in helping people to counter the contemporary concern about meaninglessness. In the previous chapter, we suggested that a concept of meaningfulness may have emerged as part of a culturally dominant set of middle class individualistic values which are rarely challenged. Christiansen (2000, p. 99) for example discussed the concept of 'personal projects' or long term goals that people saw as defining them and towards which they strived. All other activities had to be consistent with such personal projects. Furthermore, such personal projects were linked to peoples' social positions and stages in life. Thus, a young person in emerging adulthood would perhaps see establishing a career and personal position in the social world as critical personal long term goals. The youngster's daily occupations would largely be directed towards those goals. Similarly, a person who is middle aged would see helping teenage children transition to responsible adulthood and preparing for retirement as important personal projects. An older person would perhaps prioritise passing on wisdom to younger generations, and perform daily occupations in a way that would be consistent with this life project. We are hereby suggesting that meaning is somewhat linked to these important 'personal projects' which depend on socially defined roles and one's developmental stage.

In this chapter, as a first step in broadening the investigation into the characteristics of meaningful occupations, we attempt to increase comprehension of what makes occupations meaningful to people. We do this by discussing how people have tended to construct meaning in their lives using daily occupations. In one small study, Ikiugu, Pollard, Cross, et al. (2012) explored the perspectives of working class writers in the UK on meaning-making through daily occupations. The sample of 'worker-writers' autobiographies which were analysed by the researchers were drawn from a network of writing workshops, oral and community history projects, and literacy groups from various parts of the UK. This network, the Federation of Worker Writers and Community Publishers (FWWCP), was formed in 1976, and its member groups produced publications over a 30 year period. As a whole the literature produced constituted a body of knowledge about life experiences of ordinary working class people (Morley & Worpole, 2009) and provided an opportunity to help us understand how ordinary working class people use what they do on a daily basis to construct meaningful lives

(Lentin, 2002; Tatzer, van Nes & Jonsson, 2011). It formed a starting point in helping us understand how to help people in general structure their occupational performance in such a way that meaning in their lives is optimized.

In their investigation, Ikiugu et al. (2012) found that the worker-writers made meaning in their lives through common experiences found in every-day occupations. Experiences that made them feel connected to something bigger than themselves were particularly important in this meaning-making endeavour (consistent with Frankl's postulations as discussed earlier), as well as occupations that enabled individuals to persevere in occupational tasks irrespective of the barriers that they faced. The worker-writers' perceptions of how they constructed meaning using daily occupations is illustrated in figure 2-1.

As can be seen in figure 2-1, meaning in life could be visualized as a web that individuals spun throughout their lives. Unlike the web determined by an outside force such as the Norns or the sisters of fate in Norse or Greek mythology, the threads of this web were woven by the individuals for themselves. It consisted of the following: connection to something bigger than oneself; a sense of fulfilment through exploration and creativity; connection to other people, thus creating a feeling that one is not alone in the world; having a sense of social responsibility; efficacy/competence, and independence; a sense of dignity; affirmation of one's identity as an individual; making one's own life story; relevance of the experience to one's developmental stage; ability to negotiate change and adapt; ability to have intimacy through occupation; ability to transition through life; and having a place in one's cultural and temporal context that emerges from the medium of common-day experiences found in daily occupations in which individuals engage over their lifetimes.

Routes to meaning making

Through common experiences found in every-day occupations

Meaning was perceived to be a result of every day experiences emerging from daily occupational choices and performance. This finding was consistent with aspects of previous research on the relationship between occupation and meaningfulness (Christiansen, 1999; Lentin 2002; Matuska & Christiansen, 2008; Tatzer, van Nes & Jonsson, 2011). For De Certeau (1998, 1988), the common every day experiences that made life meaningful included simple things such as knowing the location of the baker's shop, knowing the geography of the street in which one lived, or understanding family recipes learned from grandmother. Thus, the theme in many of the autobiographical writings was that everyday experiences were significant, because they underpinned the social fabric in which everyone in the community shared.

Through connection to something bigger than oneself

Through common every-day experiences, many of the worker-writers felt a sense of connection to something bigger than themselves. For example, the occupation of writing and membership in the FWWCP, the organization through which they published their autobiographies, were a means of challenging the injustice within the status quo and attempting to serve a greater good. The FWWCP saw itself as a non-party based, independent, radical movement, to some extent at odds with dominant cultural perspectives, including those of other British left wing groups of the time (Morley & Worpole, 2009). The occupation of writing and membership to the FWWCP were a means of connecting personal life experiences to a larger cause. Worker-writing and the activities of the FWWCP consciously represented ordinary peoples' experiences as alternative discourses to a mainstream set of narratives which excluded it or tended to ridicule it as mundane and banal.

By a sense of fulfilment through exploration and creativity

The occupation of writing led to a sense of fulfilment for the worker-writers (Ikiugu et al., 2012), resulting from the exploration and creativity used in story-telling, and the subsequent sense of being recognized for this creative endeavour, through performance in a workshop reading, or for instance as symbolized by the book being placed on the shelves of a community bookshop. Writing from personal experiences also led to self-discovery and development of a kind of authenticity. An additional and significant element of fulfilment often arose from the process of making publications as a group and experiencing acknowledgment of these books in the community (Morley & Worpole, 2009).

By a sense of connection to others through occupation

For many of the writers, occupations contributed to meaning in life because among other things they provided a sense of connection to others in the world and made personal experiences universal. This sense of universality was achieved by individuals contributing to a shared social life through every day occupations. Thus, the topic for many of the writings was the definition of every day experiences as significant, a re-evaluation of the things that ordinary people do [occupations] because they are ordinary people, and the many little things that underpin the social fabric in which everyone shares.

This finding suggested that the relationship between identity and meaningfulness is determined by human relationships and the perceptions that people have of the ways they are viewed by others. The universality or the particularity of experience was something which was explored through social relationships and the telling and sharing of stories both within the particular context of the worker writing movement and its workshops, and in the everyday lives of the individuals who were writing the stories.

Through a sense of social responsibility

Part of what made every-day life meaningful for the worker-writers was the ability to express a sense of social responsibility. Occupations made this possible for them. Many of the writers (e.g. Beavis, 1980; Centerprise Publishing Project, 1984; Dunn 1990; Earl Marshall School, 1993; Hall, 1985; Smith 1992; Ward, 1988) discussed the contributions that they thought they made to family life or at least their part in supporting their families. Such social responsibility was sometimes expressed through actions geared towards trying to create change, such as being involved in what Kronenberg and Pollard (2005) called political activities of daily living (pADLs) through political activism or joining and being active in trade unions. This was the case for Poulsen (1988), Beckman (1992) and Sitzia and Thickett (2002) among other worker-writers.

Beavis (1980) who was a miner, Poulsen who was a Jewish worker in the tailoring trade during the 1930s, and Beckman who was one of a group of Jewish ex-servicemen confronting fascist groups in East London in the 1940s, were all examples of individuals who experienced meaning in their lives through attempts to facilitate social change for the better. For Cohen (1989), another Jewish writer, politics appeared to be attractive as a medium for change in response to Mosley's establishment of fascist headquarters in 1930s Manchester. Similarly, Thickett became politically committed after his traumatic experiences as a soldier in India during the struggle for independence and also in the Korean war (Sitzia & Thickett, 2002). Motivated by earlier experiences of hardship, he got involved in the Australian trade union movement and the campaign for aboriginal rights in the height of the cold war, and remained something of a lone activist for the rest of his life. All the above examples suggest that for the worker-writers, part of discovery of meaning in their lives involved not only reflecting on the purpose and meaning of their past occupations (such as being a British soldier during the struggle for independence in India), but also trying to make a positive contribution to society through pADLs and particularly through social activism.

Through experiences of efficacy or competence, and independence

For many years, it has been recognized in occupational therapy and occupational science literature that occupations that lead to a sense of efficacy, affirmation, and a feeling of competence in one's environment are perceived by people to be very meaningful (Abrahams, 2008; Ikiugu, 2005; Ikiugu & Rosso, 2005; Matsuka & Christiansen, 2008; Schemm & Gitlin, 1993; Schkade & Schultz, 1992; Schultz & Schkade, 1992; Seymour, 2002; Tatzer, van Nes & Jonsson, 2011). This theme was apparent in the analysis of the literature of the FWWCP writers (Ikiugu et al., 2012). Work was in particular perceived by many of the worker- writers to be a demonstration of their competency. Irrespective of how poorly it paid, work that made one feel skilful was ultimately perceived as meaningful. The majority of occupations described, for example domestic service (Noakes, 1980a; Wheway, 1984), lighterman (Harris, 1978), mining (Beavis, 1980; Moss, 1986; Muckle 1981), building work (Curley, 1993), railway guard (Ross, 1984), shop worker (Gardiner, 1985), barmaid (Barber, 1999; Tonner, 1995), agricultural work (Noakes, 1977; Scott, 1987) required specific skills. Even though many of these occupations paid relatively low wages, workers found them to be meaningful because they were a source of identity for them as skilled, competent individuals.

As an example, Harris's (1978) account demonstrated how apprenticeship accorded him status when he became a Freeman of the Watermen and Lightermen's Company in 1901. His book, written in 1935 when he was 55, was a record of the mastery of his craft, which was a source of pride for him. A good number of the other texts, for example Wren (1998), Hollick (1992), Mason

(1998), Paul (1981) and the contributors to the Centerprise working lives series (n.d., 1978) detailed the specifics about the pride of mastery through occupational performance connected to their work (for example as a taxi driver, hair dresser, or mortician).

Clearly, the *quiet pride* referred to was not always about earnings. These occupations provided validation for skills acquired over time, and it can be surmised that such skills were the source of pride for these workers in their communities. This suggests that people make meaning in their lives through the cultivation of a sense of efficacy/mastery/competence, which is sometimes symbolized by specific skills. Occupations, particularly those which are related to demonstrable skills, efficacy/mastery/competence, that can be recognised by others are important in meaning-making.

Part of this feeling of competence is the sense of independence that occupations such as work provide. As Ehn and Lofgren (2010) discovered in their discussion of Swedish rural life in the 19th century, some of the literature describes a time when there was no clear distinction between work and leisure. While it is also possible that leisure activities such as ability in sports can confer a sense of efficacy, mastery and competence, the same perception of one's abilities can also arise from simple actions. Hall (1985) contributed to the family income through occupations such as fruit picking and earned her own pocket money by cleaning out rabbit hutches and growing apples. Earning her own pocket money increased Hall's sense of independence, which was very meaningful for her. Paul (1981) felt that he attained adulthood when he was able to realize his goal of occupational performance as a craftsman. In both of these cases, a child being allowed to earn her own pocket money or a person being recognised as a skilled worker were rites of passage in which a person was recognized as having achieved a stage of development and status amongst others in the community. Finally, writing itself as an occupation was a means by which the writers' self-validation as competent people was achieved. This was consistent with Joan Erikson's (1997) remark that one of the ways in which people could evaluate their own competence was to write about it.

Through a sense of dignity

Part of the reason that occupations which fostered a sense of efficacy/competence/mastery were important for meaning making in the worker-writers' lives was because they made them feel capable and therefore dignified. Dignity is an important source of meaning in peoples' lives. Occupations, particularly work, make people feel that they have a sense of dignity. For the worker-writers, work in any form was mostly perceived to be a source of dignity. The majority of the autobiographical accounts depicted work positively or at least the individuals were presented positively as 'workers'. Such depictions included assertions of the dignity of 'work'. Sometimes even criminal activities were presented as a way of acquiring integrity. Such activities were seen as part of the experiential journey that was sometimes influenced by harsh childhood experiences, and formed a component of personal identity (Baker, 1985; Piper, 1995). This theme was represented in many ways, particularly through emphasis of forms of work that encompassed hardships. In addition, the word 'worker' was found in the titles of many of the autobiographical texts.

Through the affirmation of individual identity

A significant source of meaning for the FWWCP members as worker writers was the affirmation of their identities as individuals through their autobiographies (Ikiugu et al., 2012). The activities involving the organisation of writing and publishing were meaningful occupations because they expressed individual and community identities in terms of class and culture in a way that most people considered to be positive (Morley & Worpole, 2009; Pollard 2010; Pollard & Smart, 2012). In addition, work was for many worker-writers connected to identification with specific locations [e.g. see Dunn's (1990) *Moulsecoomb Days*, or Poulsen's (1988) *Scenes from a Stepney Youth*, Moss's (1986) *City Pit*]. Furthermore, as noted earlier, engagement in occupation was perceived to be meaningful because it was in part a means of self-discovery, and of making and telling one's life story.

In many cases, meaning making occurred in the worker-writers' lives through development of gender identity and sexual orientation. Gender-related occupations were clearly established early in the authors' lives. Many of the boyhood accounts of childhood activities involved mostly other boys (Manville, 1989, 1994; Steer, 1994), and those of the girls mostly other girls (Dunn, 1990; Masterson, 1986). In the pre-war years, school playgrounds were segregated and even some of the toys were delineated by their gender. Hall (1985) described iron hoops for boys and wooden hoops for girls. George (Brighton Ourstory Project, 1992, pp 14-15) however knew that he was gay from an early age, and described how (presumably in the late 1940s since he was born in 1936) he saved up for dolls, which he could afford to buy an arm or a leg at a time from a shop that sold doll parts. He later swapped his bike with a girl for her toy pram, to his father's consternation. His determination to possess dolls contrary to his father's wishes indicated the strength of the symbolism of occupational materials (such as dolls and toys for childhood play) in not only providing gender identity but also as an expression of sexual orientation.

If we take time to think about this simple action of exchanging a bike for a toy pram by a young man, we realize how extraordinary and important this action was. In the 1940s and 1950s, a bike or pram could have cost several pounds which would have been a substantial part of the parents' wages. Swopping these items could have caused serious trouble for the involved youngsters, because of the impression of being ungrateful to their parents. George must also have had tremendous courage and an immense motivation to risk being seen with a pram (as a boy) at this time, something that might have exposed him to community ridicule and the risk of physical violence from his peers. George's actions underscore the importance of occupations and their meaningfulness in the expression of identity.

Most of the worker-writers presented accounts of heterosexual relationships in their autobiographies. On the whole, they seemed to get married quite early in their lives. While occupations related to sexual intimacy were an element of meaning-making and identity formation in their lives, few worker-writers discussed their discovery of sexuality and related activities in much detail. Parsons (1995) took advantage of the wartime availability of groups of foreign servicemen to go dancing, while Noakes (1980a) recalled a first teenage kiss. Some parents opposed relationships on the grounds that the involved youngsters were unsuitable for their children. For example, Noakes' parents disapproved of her partner's suitability for their child, while Rose (in Padfield, 1999) expressed her disappointment with her mother for refusing to allow her to marry her first boyfriend at age 15 (although this would have been illegal in UK law). On the side of male worker-writers, Mason (1998) appeared to have been involved in some teenage sexual adventures. Daisy Noakes' husband, George, also mentioned visiting brothels during the war (Noakes, 1977).

Occupational experiences and developmental stage

The meaningfulness of everyday occupational experiences was linked to both the age of the writer at the time of writing, and the age of the person at the time of the events being described in the autobiography. At the time of the writing, most (but not all) worker-writers were reflecting on their whole working lives from the vantage point of later adult life. They described some occupational activities associated with childhood, such as apple scrumping (stealing) (Parsons 1995), the street game of 'knock down ginger', or knocking on doors and running away (Hicks 1982), fights (Manville 1994) or street battles (Wolveridge 1981) with a certain nostalgic relish. Such occupations associated with misbehaviour probably constituted rites of passage consistent with the respective childhood developmental stage described in the narrative, while they were being reflected on with the author's adult hindsight. Some writing (Millbank, 1986) took place at early adulthood. There had been a vein of more immediate writing that occurred at the inception of the FWWCP. Such autobiographical accounts were developed contemporaneously by, and with children and adolescents, and were about topics such as experiences of bullying, truancy, drug use, expression of sexuality, school, or choice of jobs. In the 1970s, these voices rarely appeared in print. Publishing schoolchildren's views on some of these 'adult' topics caused controversy because education authorities thought that this was inappropriate (Morley & Worpole, 2009).

Through ability to negotiate change and to adapt

Often worker-writers derived meaning from a sense of connection to a place: not only to the places where they lived, but also the places to which they had adapted. Work was perceived to be a means by which such connection and adaptation occurred. Thus, for Wolveridge (1981) and Muckle (1981) the 1920's depression was associated with a geographical context because its effects hit certain areas more than others. For Muckle (1981) this was due to the location of the mining industry, while for Wolveridge (1981), it was a pattern of people migrating to and settling in East London. These pockets of poverty where many people worked in the same or similar occupations were especially vulnerable to economic changes.

Occupations themselves symbolised the worker-writers' experiences of change. Older writers recorded differences in their work practices alongside social changes that had occurred throughout their lifetimes. Many worker writers noted improvement in work conditions, the effects of urbanisation, or they recorded the disappearance of community features. They also described enduring harsh life experiences arising from previous social attitudes, such as childhood punishment that may be described today as child abuse (Masterson, 1986; Dalley, 1998), including being caned to correct left-handedness (Hall, 1985), racial and sexual abuse (Wiltshire, 1985) or nearly dying from influenza due to inability to afford medicine in the period before state health services became available (Healey, 1980).

Occupations that seemed to be the most important for daily meaning-making were those that had survival value because they were a means of adapting to difficult circumstances. The worker-writers frequently discussed the cost of household goods and food and the various means their parents used to make do. Carter's (1992) butcher's apprentice brother brought unsellable offal home so that the family could use it to make stew. Masterson's (1986) family on the other hand had to eat their pet rabbit, having nothing else for Christmas dinner. Hall's (1985) father killed a rook who was stealing their potatoes, and the culprit was made into a pie by her mother. Capstick (1988) described the rediscovery of these adaptive skills in more recent times of hardship (as illustrated during the 1972 miners' strike), such as using caramelised sugar heated in a spoon to make gravy browning, a technique her grandmother had taught her early in her life. This adaptation occurred in areas other than food as well: for example, Barnes (1976) learned from his dad to stuff his bicycle tyres with newspapers because he could not afford inner tubes.

Occupations whose meaningfulness was associated closely with the negotiation of change and adaptation often marked the rites of passage mentioned earlier in this chapter. One example which many worker-writers described was entering the world of work. This rite of passage marked a transition from a state of childhood to that of responsible adulthood. Working life appeared for many to be the point at which most childlike things and occupations were left behind. The autobiographies covered a period in which there were notable changes in the UK age of school termination from 13 to 16. Wren (1998) for example began his autobiography by describing his experience of leaving school at age 14 so that he could begin his wartime apprenticeship, thus taking up the responsibility of an adult citizen. In many of the earlier accounts, the autobiographers transitioned straight from school to work, often taking jobs that were arranged for them by their parents.

Other writers described social barriers to age-appropriate tasks that made transition difficult, thus creating a sense of meaninglessness. For example, writers with disability experienced many barriers to acquiring gainful employment. When Millbank (1986) left school, she found that the careers service could only refer her to social services. It took three years for her to find sheltered employment. Wiltshire (1985) was persecuted by her family and their friends, and was unable to find work while living in Jamaica in the late 1960s and 1970s. Eventually she moved to England where she thought that people with disability would be better protected in the hope of getting a job, but only experienced further abuse.

Through intimacy-related occupations

Another marker of the transition from childhood for many worker-writers was marriage. Erikson, (1997, p. 70) described marriage as a transition in which individuals were launched into adulthood through the formation of relationships where 'work, sexuality and friendship promised to prove complementary.' Despite the importance of intimate relationships in the meaning-making process for these worker-writers, there were some aspects of intimacy which proved difficult to negotiate. Marriage was not available to the gay contributors to *Daring Hearts* (Brighton Ourstory Project, 1992). For them independence or even a complete break from family members had to be achieved before relationships could be established safely without the threat of disruption by public, legal, and family interventions. The contributors found it hard to express themselves, trust people, build relationships, and construct their lives in the community in a censorious and oppressive society. As a consequence of this insecurity, as one of the autobiographers stated, 'everybody in the gay scene, I suppose, they all seem to be searching, searching and looking' (Peter, Brighton Ourstory Project, 1992, p. 40).

Many of the accounts of early married life during that time consisted of descriptions of material hardships. As titles such as *Hard work and no consideration* (Paul, 1981) suggest, many of the worker-writers saw their lives in that period as consisting of poverty and hard life. Noakes (1980b) described how her husband had to go back to work the day after their wedding and the poor living conditions in their early years of marriage. She was unprepared for the isolation which went with housework, which was made worse by her husband George's habit of reading the paper at the meal table. Both of them were to negotiate and come to a compromise regarding how to communicate better. One of their occupation-based solutions was for her husband to teach her a card game in the evenings so that they would have a social activity in which they could engage together.

Another event that impacted on the meaning of marriage and intimacy was the second World War, which offered opportunities for couples to develop a kind of constrained intimacy. Dunn (1990) and Smith (1992) got married while their partners were briefly on leave from service in the war. Davey (1980) discussed the lack of privacy in her early married life due to the forced living environment in single rented rooms, often shared with her mother in law. At one point she returned to her mother in Yorkshire where she lived until her husband was released from the military base in London to be with her.

In all these accounts, it seems that couples developed intimacy by making accommodations (Erikson, 1997) or occupational adaptations to deal with tough life circumstances. Beavis (1980) rented two rooms for himself and his new wife from a friend, initially content to furnish them with an old bed, a chest of drawers and an orange box covered with a curtain. Ward (1988), who also got married during the war, eventually got her first home after the birth of her daughter. Although she was able to furnish much of it, there was only *one camp chair in the living room* (the title of her book). She and her husband had to take turns sitting on it.

Through a sense of belonging in one's culture and temporal context

The worker-writers seemed to conceive the development of their identities as occurring within the context of place and occupations, including work and time. Of those autobiographies that were analysed by Ikiugu et al. (2012), 31 referred to place [or distance from home in the case of some of the books by migrants (Adams, 1987; Akter, 1998)]. Other autobiographies referred to cultural experiences (e.g. Centerprise, 1984; Ethnic Communities Oral History Project, 1993). Clearly, for these worker-writers, there were relationships among occupation, social context, historical context, and geographical community.

The meaning of occupational contextualization also included a temporal (historical) component. For example, by the time Moss (1986) wrote his autobiography, the Bristol based city pit to which his narrative referred had been closed. Similar memories of childhood were also evoked by Wheway (1984), Hall (1985), and Cook (1983). The title of Manville's (1989) autobiography, *Everything seems smaller*, illustrated this difference between the past and the present. The fact that the temporal and spatial contexts of past occupations were a source of identity for the writers was clear from the example of the community publishing group, QueenSpark (Morley & Worpole, 2009). QueenSpark's series of books, some of which were analysed in the Ikiugu et al's (2012) study, had been developed from a community newspaper column in which there had been much interest in representing the history of the area by local people. Some writers were motivated to make their contributions by reading the pieces other people had written. Many of the authors were therefore writing for people like themselves, in an attempt to trigger memories in others as well as to speak to younger generations. As an example, Carter (1992) referred his readers to Manville (1989) for a description of the street games that he used to play as a child.

In other texts the worker-writers frequently referred to specific streets, shops, places of work and recreation and the people who would have been found in those places. These references were meant to be understood and recognised by a local readership, in a written form of what De Certeau et al. (1998) called a micro-history. In some of the shorter contributions to *Bristol Lives* (Bristol

Broadsides, 1987) and *More Bristol Lives* (Bristol Broadsides, 1988) these details were the main focus of the authors' autobiographies. Many QueenSpark authors also gave careful accounts of local geography. Manville's accounts (1989, 1994) for instance exemplified this contextualization of occupations. He carefully identified both location and incidence to illustrate his boyhood preoccupation with the consumption of 'broken' goods (shop refuse which could be sweets, chocolate, or biscuits), or attending cinemas. A sense of place, time, and social environment provided these writers with strong contexts for their narratives of occupational lives. In these narratives, they articulated their sense of belonging to particular communities through doing, being, and becoming (e.g. Marshall, 1984; Mason, 1998; Monaf, 1994; Poulsen, 1988).

The meaning associated with place was even more critical for authors whose origins were outside the UK (Adams, 1987; Earl Marshall School, 1993; Ethnic Communities Oral History Project, 1993; Gordon, 1985; Wiltshire 1985). These autobiographers described the contrasts between the environments in which they had grown up and those to which they had migrated, sometimes forcefully. For example, Fozia (Earl Marshall School, 1993, pp. 127-131) gave a compelling account of how she escaped massacre in Northern Somalia during the civil war in the 1980's. Others tried to make sense of their lives by adapting to their new environments through pursuit of work opportunities in the UK. In Adams (1987) Islam and Qureshi described how they went about establishing some of the first Indian restaurants in the UK during the 1920s and 1930s, initially to cater for their own migrant community. The 'Indian' cuisine which developed from such pioneering occupational engagements has since become popularised as a major part of the British cuisine and cultural heritage.

Other authors from the Caribbean (e.g. Noble, 1984; Wilshire, 1985) described their struggles in the process of settling down in the UK. Establishing life in a new community and engaging in new occupations presented a range of challenges to immigrant worker-writers, not only because of the negative experiences of racism and violence, but also because of the expectations placed on them by their relatives back home. In the UK they experienced occupational deprivation which probably made them feel doubtful about their sense of purpose. This was illustrated best by Gordon (1985) who described his attempts to explain to his Jamaican neighbours that moving to the UK had not made him wealthier either materially or occupationally. His income was barely enough for rent, tax, and maintenance of a second hand car. The fruits and vegetables that his wife bought at the market were of a standard that people back home would not even bother to pick. While Gordon's perception was that his standard of living had declined in many important respects, he was identified by his Jamaican friends and relatives as well off because of his migration to the UK.

Gordon's experiences indicated that a large component of occupational identity (and by extension, meaning in life) is likely to be based on occupational performance, but this performance is affected by social or technological changes, or migration to different cultural environments. Even though people learn to adapt, their present sense of doing, being, becoming and belonging affects their experience of adaptation and in turn is incorporated into their identity.

Conclusion

As the analysis of the autobiographies of the English members of the FWWCP by Ikiugu et al. (2012) indicated, experiences in every day occupations are important raw material that human beings use to create meaning in their lives. Through such occupations, individuals are able to establish a durable identity for themselves, connect to other people so that they do not feel alone, connect to a cause that is bigger than themselves, recognize their transitions through life and adaptation to changes, explore and experience a sense of creativity, have a sense of dignity, and feel connected to their temporal and spatial contexts. These themes illuminate the possibilities of developing strategies to help people confront the meaninglessness that Frankl (1969) identified as a problem in modern life. Occupational therapy and occupational science have the potential to facilitate deeper exploration of meaning in peoples' lives using such themes as guidelines in occupation-based interventions to confront the problem of meaninglessness. We will return to these ideas in subsequent chapters.

Applying the ideas discussed in Chapter 2

In chapter one, you guided your client to rate himself in regards to his sense of meaning in life and the things that he thought made life meaningful. After reading chapter two, continue the exploration of that theme by identifying the common experiences in every-day occupations that your client thinks contribute to a sense of meaning in his life. Following are some exercises that may help with this process of reflection and exploration:

1. Helping the client realize how every-day occupational experiences create meaning

Favourite recipes. Meals and recipes are a basic part of a person's everyday routine. Many people have a favourite food that reminds them of a person, a place, or something important, perhaps particular events in their lives. Ask your client to think about such meals and why they might be important. Whether it is something the client makes, or somebody else makes it for her or whether the client cooks it from scratch or just pops it in the microwave, have her think about the steps followed in preparing and enjoying this food. Perhaps there is a particular smell, perhaps the food ingredients are found on a particular shelf in the supermarket, or the client eats the food from a particular plate. Now have the client imagine that this food is no longer available. How would that lack impact her life? Does she need to replace the food or meal experience with something else, and if so what? Have the client write down her reflections and discuss them with you.

2. Helping the client realize how meaning can be maintained through transitions by adapting to change

Changing jobs. With increasing flexibility in the modes of production, most people are going to experience a career change at least once in their lives. These changes require the ability to transition and to adapt to new ways of engaging in productive occupations. Now, ask your client to tell you about his work. Have aspects of his job tasks already been incorporated into another job role occupied by someone else, or has his job been eliminated for any reason? If so, what changes did your client make, or what is your client planning to do, in order to continue to work? If a change has not occurred, ask the client to imagine that his present job has become obsolete and the duties in that job have been assimilated into another work role. Have the client write down or imagine what he might say about himself if he were seeking a new position at a job agency and is interviewing for the job, *but without using the title of his current job, or of a job that has already become obsolete.* It may help for the client to use stems such as the following in the statements: 'I can…'; 'I am…'; 'People perceive me as…'

3. Helping the client become clear about personal identity

Origins. Ask your client to answer the following question: 'Where am I from?' Most people identify themselves with a place and possibly a time in which they grew up. Ask your client to draw a family tree and describe the context of growing up. One key to this reflection might be for the client to try and remember the stories parents and grandparents told her about previous generations in the family. What memories does your client hold, that define for her whom she is? Another approach might be for the client to imagine earliest memories of walking out of home to visit specific places in the neighbourhood: the corner shop; the school; friends' homes. What features along the way can the client remember? Ask her to compare each of these features to those in a place that she currently frequents as a way of improving awareness of place and time in which she exists.

4. Helping the client to become aware of how connection to other people enhances meaning in life

Familiar words. Nearly all people have an idiolect, a unique use of language developed in communication with friends and family, as well as a dialect which relates to the wider community in which they live. What particular words has your client developed, or what words does he choose to use to talk about familiar objects and actions that perhaps are unique and different from the words that other people use? Common examples might be the words that people use for types of bread (e.g. roll, bap, barmcake, cob, teacake, breadcake, bun - all of which are potentially similar but may refer to quite different forms of bread in the regional dialects of the UK), types of sweets/candy, or vegetables. Why are those words important to your client? How do the words (or did in the past) help the client connect with significant people in his life? Why are/were those connections important? Have the client reflect on these questions and write down the answers.

5. Helping the client enhance meaning in life by being aware of personal identity

Personal objects. Ask your client to tell you a story about using five objects that are personally significant to her. The client can develop a slide show of these objects as part of therapeutic intervention and do a presentation, or perhaps photograph them and share them through a smart phone. In each slide or picture, ask her to explain the object (what it is and where it came from), as well as its part and the meaning it provides to her life story, and whom she perceives herself to be. What does your client think that these objects signify about her (both positive and negative qualities), or any changes that she might want to make in her life?

Chapter 3
The human quest for meaning

Learning Objectives

By the end of this chapter, the reader will demonstrate an understanding of:

1. The search for meaning as a perennial human endeavor
2. How human beings use cultural, religious, and intellectual institutions as a means of pursuing life meaning
3. The institutional (cultural, religious, and intellectual) means by which human beings pursue meaning in life
4. How people in general can be helped to explore ways of optimizing/enriching their search for meaning in life through daily occupations in the context of cultural, religious, and intellectual institutions

Contents of this chapter

- Cultural institutions as tools for definition of occupational meaning
- Religion and other cultural traditions such as myths, legends, and folklore as a way of comprehending the world and making it meaningful
- Intellectual pursuits as symbolic vehicles in the quest for meaning through attempts to tell the story of 'how we chose to be what we became'

The search for meaning as a perennial human quest

According to one of the most accepted definitions in the profession of occupational science and occupational therapy, meaningful occupation refers to ordinary and familiar things that people do, that are: personally meaningful; age appropriate; and *accepted in one's culture;* including things that people do for self-maintenance (self-care), productivity (work, volunteering, home management, etc.), and leisure (American Occupational Therapy Association [AOTA], 2014; Ikiugu, 2007; Law, Polatajko, Baptiste, & Townsend, 2002). We highlight the "accepted in one's culture" part of this definition to emphasize the fact that the meaningfulness that individuals derive from participation in occupations is to a large extent culturally determined. Therefore, it is important that as occupational therapists and scientists, we examine cultural institutions that define the meaning of occupations for human beings.

As mentioned in Chapter 1, throughout history, human beings have thought about the meaning of their existence. According to Wolpert (2007) the quest for the meaning of existence began with an ingrained human desire to understand. It started with insight into cause and effect relationships between events, which in turn led to development of tools. In essence, Wolpert seems to agree in principle with the originator of the philosophy of pragmatism, Charles Sanders Peirce (1955), who postulated that the human mind finds tranquility in belief, while doubt causes discomfort which has to be resolved by re-establishing belief.

Once our ancestors had developed tools, they started experiencing themselves as causes. They could see the cause and effect relationships between their actions and consequences, and were therefore able to explain those consequences. It is widely supposed that from this point on, human beings felt compelled to explain other life mysteries, including issues of life and death (Fernandez-Armesto, 2001; Schama, 1995; Wolpert, 2007). In this endeavor they conceived of gods and spirits to explain the regulation of those natural events that were out of their control and which could not be explained easily. Even though such gods and spirits could not be seen, their influence could be evidenced in the course of nature. Thus a fundamental connection was established between belief and the human struggle for survival. Over the course of evolution, spiritual knowledge became a significant source of meaning for human beings. In this chapter, the human quest for meaning will be explored by examining the role of culturally determined belief-supporting institutions in meaning-making in human life. In many respects the quest for meaning through belief-supporting institutions can be seen historically not only as an attempt to explain natural phenomena but also as what Marr (2007, p. xxvi) described as the story of 'how we chose to be what we became'. In the chapter we will discuss religion as well as wider cultural traditions, myths, legends, and folk-tales, and intellectual pursuits as symbolic vehicles that many people use in their quest for meaning and in their attempts to tell the story of 'how we chose to be what we became'.

Legends, myths, and folklore are important means of communicating shared aspects of culture (Jones, 1995). Myths are stories which attempt to explain the origin of the world or people, or to explain how nature works and how people should treat each other. Legends are based on historical accounts of people and their actions, but the facts are changed to make the story interesting, convincing, or inspiring. For example, the story about how the Meru people of Kenya were enslaved in a place called Mbwaa by the 'red people' is a myth (although there are indications that it could be referring to the enslavement of the Bantu people by the Arabs in the East African island of Zanzibar) which attempts to explain the origin of the Meru people (Finke, 2003). On the other hand stories about how Mwariama and Dedan Kimathi could transform themselves into animal forms in order to infiltrate the British troops during the 'Mau Mau' struggle for the Kenyan independence from the British are legends (Jamuhuri Team, 2012). Mwariama and Kimathi were actually generals who led the Mau Mau warriors. However, they were mere human beings and did not really have the supernatural powers attributed to them in the legends.

Folktales and folk lore are situated in the everyday lives of a group of people. Today folk tales are mostly understood as fictional or fantastical stories whose magical characters such as goblins, elves, and giants are usually used to teach children specific moral lessons about life. Folk stories and other forms of folk lore are essentially oral, and their themes are repeated through many cultures. However, the commonly held idea that they were made exclusively for children has only emerged since they were written down. They were and still are addressed to an adult audience and new stories are emerging all the time, as much in modern society as in pre-literary ones.

These stories often have a function, which is to define the boundaries of group membership, and to serve as vehicles for social participation, for example when they are used in telling jokes, or in group story-telling, or in participatory folk songs. Legends, myths and folktales are all creations of the collective human mind encapsulating a popular sense of ethics, principles and cultural aspirations, combining new and obscurely ancient elements. They are a part of every human society, and can circulate very rapidly. As such, they are an important set of cultural vehicles for the expression of life meaning.

For occupational therapists and occupational scientists, it is important to cultivate a deeper understanding of how culture relates to meaning in human lives. First, as mentioned in chapter one, the existential vacuum defined by Frankl (1992) can be understood as resulting from loss of human connection with nature, traditions, religion, and other belief-supporting institutions described by Wolpert (2007) and others. This disconnectedness has been identified by some as the underlying cause of the 2011 riots in the UK, taking the form of erosion in self-discipline, lack of adequate leadership for the youth, and alienation of the youth from society (British Broadcasting Corporation [BBC], 2012). Ivanov (2011) suggested that the British riots and the wave of Arab Spring uprisings in the Middle East shared similar features such as social exclusion and the fracturing of society leading to a rise in levels of poverty and desperation. Numerous socialist political thinkers and social reformers were making similar points during the 19th century. Social disparity gave rise to the initial development of the occupational therapy profession (Frank, 1992; Frank & Zemke, 2008). Experience and knowledge of social differences and inequality in occupational opportunity and choice is a consistent theme in culture, a point underscored by the finding in chapter two that the English worker-writers' meaning-making in part emerged from engaging in occupations that were part of their occupational identities and facilitated their sense of cultural belonging. Culture is an important repository for a community's beliefs and traditions. Individuals seek opportunities to engage in occupations that connect them meaningfully to these existential traditions.

This connectedness to existential traditions through occupational performance is important to occupational therapists and occupational scientists as indicated by the current attempts in the two disciplines to identify situations where people are denied access to meaningful and purposeful occupations, resulting in occupational deprivation (Whiteford, 2000). Frankl's (1992) concept of *noogenic neurosis* is based in part on the assumption that people who experience meaninglessness tend to have lost their connection to valued work. One of the services that occupational therapists and scientists can offer to society is to help such people reconnect with their beliefs and traditions through engagement in culturally valued occupations.

How human beings use cultural, religious, and intellectual institutions as a means of pursuing life meaning

The definition of culture has changed over human history. According to Williams (1976) the English use of the word 'culture' was originally connected with the cultivation of plants and rearing of animals necessary for survival. In other words, 'culture' developed from human beings settling down in agricultural communities. From the 16th century, the meaning of the word culture was extended to refer to 'human development', and eventually came to mean 'civilization'. However, Williams cited the German philosopher Herder as having used the word to refer to a way of life. In the 20th century, culture continued to be associated with human development as expressed in constructs such as 'civilization', while it also came to refer to intellectual, artistic, and spiritual matters. As an anthropological term, culture is a recent conceptualization.

In recent times, culture has also been seen as a resource, used to enable cultural insiders to succeed socially (and even economically) over outsiders. Bourdieu (1986) coined the concept of cultural capital, which referred to the assumption that formalised knowledge received through education endows the privileged members of society (cultural insiders) with rights that may be unavailable to others (outsiders). This advantageous position of individuals occurs through specific enculturation programmes (e.g. education that leads to recognition of skills through certification) which lead to placement of the individuals into higher social status. In some cases, culture may confer advantage to individuals by birth. In the 18th and 19th centuries, aristocratic birth was often associated with high culture and privilege (Williams, 1976), perhaps because the social process of acquiring culture was often made possible through the wealth and privileges afforded by social class. Even in modern society, membership to privileged classes is often achieved through birth into a wealthy family. Clearly, there is a relationship between wealth, the attendance of elite educational institutions, and positions of power for many individuals.

But what is culture in essence? Anthropologists Bates and Plog (1990, p. 7) defined it as "a system of shared beliefs, values, customs, behaviors, and artifacts that the members of a society use to cope with their world and with one another, and that are transmitted from generation to generation through learning". This definition implies that culture has the following important characteristics:

1. It is all encompassing, involving everything that human beings do in their business of living. This includes not only values, beliefs, and opinions that people hold, but also their industry, technology, and products.

2. It is a tool for adaptation. Culture makes it possible for a group of people to "cope with their world". Therefore, it is an existential phenomenon. In our definition of meaningfulness, we proposed that things that are most meaningful to people may be those that are related to their survival (i.e. have existential value). Already, we can see why culture is such an important conveyer of human beings on their quest for life meaning. It is related to their survival and therefore meets the existential criterion of the definition of meaningfulness.
3. It is the basis for interpersonal communication. Culture makes meaningful interactions among members of a society possible. As Williams (1976, p. 78) stated, the epistemological root of the word culture is "cultivation", which alludes to its origin in "agriculture". It is only after human beings settled in agricultural communities that cultural mores evolved as a means of regulating communication and interactions among individuals in the community. These mores were communicated by community members to each other and enabled them to respond to environmental demands effectively and therefore to adapt.
4. Finally, culture is a learned phenomenon. It is transmitted from generation to generation through some form of education. In traditional societies, this transmission was by oral instruction. Today, there are formalized education systems through which culture is learned although some aspects of it are still transmitted orally, informally, and through modeling (for example the forms of dressing that are considered appropriate in different cultural settings, hunting activities, and the social rituals that are adopted by communities as leisure activities). Many of the everyday practices which define the culture of occupational therapy are for example inculcated through oral transmission (Detweiler & Peyton, 1999).

Given this all-inclusive definition, it is clear that culture grounds people in their communities by providing them with a collective identity as a group. In chapter two, we discussed the sense of connection to others that emerged as a strong theme in meaning-making by English worker-writers. These narratives demonstrated how particular cultural artifacts, practices, and ways of life were profoundly meaningful, because they defined the way that members of a community could express their shared belonging in the community. Tevye, the central protagonist in the movie "*Fiddler on the Roof*" stated this most aptly when he pointed out that culture is a means of helping people maintain their balance (and capacity for survival). In the film, Tevye used the metaphor of a fiddler trying to balance on the roof while playing his instrument as an analogy for the stabilizing role of traditions. The title of the film comes from Tevye's statement that without traditions, he (and his people) would be "as shaky as a fiddler on the roof".

Religion as a vehicle in the quest for meaning

Religion is one of the enduring and most important elements of culture that serves a grounding function. Although religious institutions have had to adjust to technological innovations and resulting social change, religious expression has remained tied largely to unchanging texts, even if interpretations of the texts have changed significantly over time. For many people, religion may be seen as an institution with a pragmatic purpose related to human survival. Evolutionary biologists such as Dawkins (2008) and Wolpert (2007) suggest that while religion is a dangerous delusion considering the suffering caused by religious believers over the course of human history, it may be a tool used by humans to adapt to their environments. As Dawkins (2010) suggested, the evolutionary value of religion may have been and still may be in the psychological protection that it provides, just like a child who obeys an elder's advice not to touch a snake may be protected from the snake-bite and possible death. The value is not in any assumption of supernatural powers of the advice, but in the pragmatic consequences that could result from following the advice. For example, if a person is extremely annoyed by another person to the point of desiring to seriously harm that individual, but obeys the commandment not to kill, the result would be that he would be protected from committing murder, and the potential victim may be protected from possible death. The value of this eventuality is not necessarily in the belief that if he had killed the offending person he would burn in hell, but in the fact that the life in question is preserved, and thus chances of preserving the human gene-pool in general are increased. If that is the case, then religion has existential value and therefore participation in religious practices provides meaning in life specifically for that purpose. For others (Barr, 1992; Wilson, 2005) the real meaning of religion is in its transcendental function in helping people get closer to: attainment of eternal bliss; salvation of souls; and deliverance of people to heaven rather than solving the problems of this world.

The story of Adam and Eve in the Garden of Eden is one of the key stories in the Judeo-Christian tradition that reveals how religion is related to meaning in life. Barr (1992) suggested that this was a story about the development of knowledge, and the recognition of mortality that came with the loss of innocence. Eve was persuaded through cunning (by the serpent) to eat of the tree of knowledge, involved Adam, and consequently they had to leave the garden in which everything had come naturally. Instead they had to till the soil to survive, and occupy and domesticate territory, thereby establishing the whole basis for what occupational therapists and scientists might term occupational performance, paving the way for subsequent constructs of occupational justice, and injustice. The story was probably a figurative description of the transition from hunting and gathering to settlement in early attempts to cultivate the land. The bible story continued to explain how descendants of Adam and Eve's son Cain advanced human social development further by building the first city. This was probably a description of another transition from agricultural based communities to urbanization, which resulted in new problems.

By evolving from a natural state of innocence to an awareness of their condition as humans, Adam and Eve had to work in an attempt to exploit the land by extracting the needed resources, and to defend their way of life from threats (evil) that they had not known in the natural state of the garden. Knowledge of good also entailed knowledge of evil. The transition from an innocent and natural state to this kind of awareness is something that both distinguishes humans from other animals (since they can know a God and are, unlike beasts, conceived in his image), and at the same time entails a recognition that humans are no different from other animals because they die as every other living thing dies. At the same time the knowledge of death perhaps led to a sense of the eternal and the hope that it may somehow be possible to evade mortality. Without any human technical means to ensure attainment of immortality, a solution was found in recognition of God as a mediator of access to the eternity of heaven. After all, as Barr (1992) pointed out, once he had been expelled from the garden, Adam was too busy with everyday toil to develop other capacities, so he had to leave many things to God.

For many devout believers, the transcendental function of faith is the true meaning of religious affiliation. Contemplation of the after-life is the vehicle to ultimate meaning for them. However, even in their transcendental orientation, many religions still take mundane reality into account and recognize a value in it. Pargament (2008, p. 23) for example equated spirituality and religion with what he referred to as "the sacred", at the core of which" lie perceptions of God, divinity, and transcendent reality". However, he saw this sacred as being revealed in all the events of our daily reality. In other words, in Pargament's view, the sacred is:

1. manifested in our daily lives;
2. transcendent or "boundless" and involves "the perception of endless time and space" (p. 24); and
3. constitutes the ultimate truth.

Thus, he saw the sacred as defining the conditions under which daily activity took place. The sacred suggested a greater continuity than is perceptible in an individual life, because it allowed for the expression of a shared purpose among individuals, groups, and generations. Through the continuity of endless time and space, it had a holding function, one which deferred individual needs to the service of a higher order or truth. For people in the Judeo Christian tradition this concept of the sacred denotes connection to something larger than oneself, as we discussed in chapter two. However, this concept may also be expressed in terms other than through relationship to a deity. It may for example refer to the universe, to the spirits of ancestors, or some process of enlightenment. It may even refer to affiliation to an organization that is committed to solution of important global problems, such as a political party, an environmental movement, etc. For evolutionists, there are four ways of explaining how religion originated (Wilson, 2005), which gives us an inkling as to why it is such an important conveyance for individuals in their search for meaning.

According to Wilson, there are four ways of understanding the role of religion in human life:

1. Religion can be understood to have evolved as a means of group adaptation. It conferred an advantage to groups over their competitors so that members of those groups with religion were able to survive and reproduce, and therefore dominate the human gene pool;
2. Religious practices helped individuals adapt. In this way, religion benefited individuals (primarily leaders) within groups;
3. In agreement with Dawkins (2008), Wilson concedes that there is a possibility that religion evolved as a cultural parasite whose purpose was to enable cultures to maintain control over individuals. In this view, religion may be understood purely as a means by which cultural power was exerted over individuals, and this was the whole purpose of religion, and there was no other functional value;
4. Another view is that religion is really a by-product of traits (such as thinking processes) that helped human beings adapt to demands of non-religious contexts, but it is not adaptive in itself. For example, the cost-benefit thinking that is so beneficial in economics and the notion of bargaining as a way of maximizing benefits led to an attempt to bargain for other benefits that are beyond the reach of people, such as a long life, good health, rainfall, or a bountiful harvest. If people were not able to produce such benefits by their own efforts, it followed that the benefits had to be gifts from a higher power to whom appeals could be made for more of the gifts. Such a higher power often resided in some conspicuous feature of the landscape such as a stone, a bush, etc. In this sense, according to Dawkins, religion was a byproduct of the adaptive economic thinking, in which human beings attempted to make a deal with the higher being that they called God, as a way of maximizing their advantages on this earth and beyond.

The most comprehensive elucidation of the evolutionary value of religion as a vehicle in the quest for meaning was that by Wilson (2002) and Wilson, van Vugt, and O'Gorman (2008). Wilson developed what he termed the Multilevel Selection (MLS) theory as a way of explaining religion as a means of group selection. In this theory, social groups were postulated to have evolved through what he referred to as a higher level selection (Wilson, 2005, 2002). He proposed that altruistic groups tended to survive more effectively than those that were less altruistic, giving them dominance in the human gene pool. In other words, when a group's altruistic characteristics superseded its members' individualistic selfish tendencies, this higher level selection enabled the entire group to adapt more successfully and therefore to thrive. A contemporary illustration of the value of altruism is the relative prosperity and stability of democratic societies over other societies in which egalitarian equality is less emphasized. Of course we have to remember that many complex interacting factors such as geography, climate, and the availability of resources also play a part in this evolutionary process.

In Wilson's (2008) MLS theory, the formation of groups as adaptive units characterized a major transition for early human beings. This was the point at which people developed the ability to form groups that acted like super-organisms composed of individuals functioning analogically like organs in a biological body. This major evolutionary transition enabled those in the groups to adapt to varying environmental conditions and thus colonize the entire world. Between-group selection dominated as social groups became higher level organisms coalescing into larger and larger entities. Groups in which there was cohesion, enabling them to maintain super-organism status, had a survival advantage over individuals and uncoordinated groups. Altruism was a very important mechanism for maintaining such cohesiveness.

Wilson (2007, p. 3 of 4) further argued that: "Groups of individuals who possess these [altruistic] capacities survive and reproduce better than groups that don't." If a society experiences loss of social cohesion and social capital, its altruistic tendencies could be diminished, hurting human chances of survival in the long term. People belonging to such a society may consequently experience increasing meaninglessness. What Frankl (1992) called *noogenic neurosis* could therefore be a symptom of a sick society that has moved away from the social genetic structure in which the building block is empathy and altruism. The recent global economic crisis, the looming catastrophe precipitated by the climate change, and the scarcity of certain raw materials are the by-products of human occupational activity that could be seen as an expression of other symptoms of this illness of a society whose genetic building blocks have mutated from altruism (normal state of a healthy society) to radical individualism (a sick society). As the sense of altruism becomes lost and people become reluctant to make the sacrifices necessary to address the problems facing us collectively, despite recognizing the evident effects they are having, they are choosing to serve their interests at the expense of collective well-being and perhaps of posterity. These actions may actually be pushing the human species towards a crisis and possible eventual self-extinction. To reverse this course, enough people have to recognise the benefits of reciprocity, i.e. developing the empathy needed to change their behavior and to trust each other for their actions to be effective.

In other words, the altruistic mechanism does not only serve a moral but a practical purpose of maintaining an equilibrium that is necessary for human survival as a species. People in many hunter-gatherer societies understood that it was necessary to move on to allow the ecology to recover and to ensure a constant and varied food supply. This understanding was clear in their respect for the spirits of the animals and plants upon which they depended. Actions such as asking permission of an animal to hunt it, or of the tree to yield its fruit were small ceremonies which enabled decisions to be made about the appropriateness of the prey or the harvest from a forest in which the hunters regarded themselves as guests (Smith, 1980). It was a way of preserving resources for use by everybody as well as for use by posterity. They knew that if a group of people killed too many animals, especially females which were responsible for propagating the animal species, or over-harvested a certain type of food, the stock would be depleted in that area precipitating a shortage in the following year. Seeking permission from the prey was a way of being mindful of the needs of all, and was therefore beneficial to the survival of both the people and the environment on which they depended.

From the ensuing discussion, it can be inferred that the development of religious and cultural moral codes provided control mechanisms to reign in selfishness and establish the trust which was essential for groups to form and stay together – though notice that Dawkins (2006) was very skeptical of this view, preferring the genetic theory of selfishness and self-preservation rather than altruism. Where there was trust, people were able to find meaning and reward in their group identity, making it attractive to choose co-operation with others rather than to be in conflict with others. In time, preference for "altruism, benevolence, retaliation, contrition, fairness, forgiveness, and so on" (Wilson et al., 2008, p. 7) became a human evolutionary trait. Religious and cultural morality made the attainment of these preferences possible.

Wilson (2008) argued that because altruism was so advantageous to group survival, motivation for altruistic actions, or moral direction, was also part of human evolution since it encouraged group cohesiveness. In other words, as Hurd (2004, p. 152) stated, the true purpose of religion was "really about encouraging altruism within the group to enable the social unit to thrive". Furthermore, religion provided human beings with the ability to keep going when things became difficult because it instilled hope and faith in the absence of information about how events might turn out. With this hope came the ability to delay gratification, and to forgive others, both characteristics that enable not only groups but also individuals to adapt. Thus whether one believes in the mystical transcendental realities postulated by religious faiths, such as eternal life, heaven and hell, God, and angels, or in the evolutionary utilitarian value of religion, it can be argued that religion is an institution through which many people have pursued meaning for ages, because it has an existential survival value.

Cultural imagination as a means to meaning: The role of myths and legends

In their quest for meaning, human beings in every culture have engaged in the imaginative activity of mythology, folktales and legends. Many of these creations of their collective minds are understandably related to religious conceptions since they originate from the same source; the supernatural, imaginative, magical explanation of the meaning of existence. Some authors suppose that these stories represent the collective aspirations of a community and are and expression of their collective soul (Chiriac, 2007). Often, this mythical quest for meaning is represented by heroes who confront the unknown, thereby dramatizing the human existential desire to create, destroy, explore, rejuvenate, and inhabit the world (Peterson, 2000). The hero in such tales represents not only a people's ideals but also their aspirations (Chiriac, 2007).

In order to be meaningful, the heroic quest is often characterized by struggle, where the hero engages in a dangerous confrontation (always for altruistic rather than selfish purposes, such as saving a loved one, saving humanity, etc.) and eventually triumphs. For example, in Greek mythology, the Titan Prometheus loved human beings very much (because he had created them). He tricked Zeus into accepting the portion of a bull sacrifice which contained the bones and fat, concealing the flesh so that men could have it. On discovering his deception Zeus declared that men could eat the flesh but they had to eat it raw. Prometheus persuaded Athene, Zeus's daughter, to let him into Mount Olympus to steal fire from the sun chariot so that he could give it to humankind (Forbush, 1928; Graves, 1960). The implication of the story, which is possibly one of the earliest narratives depicting humanity's origins, is that Prometheus gave people not only fire, but the skills to make it. The gift of Prometheus was in effect the gift of technology, of the means of developing crafts and professions that enabled humans to develop a civilization (Fernandez-Armesto, 2000).

When Zeus saw that human beings had fire, he was angry and ordered Prometheus to be bound with iron chains to the side of a wild and stormy Caucasus mountain, and sent a vulture to gnaw at his heart (or in some versions his liver) every day. Prometheus was a Titan, one of a race of immortal gods who preceded Zeus and the other Olympians. Unable to die, he suffered in silence for many years. In this legend, one can see parallels to the story of Jesus, not only because of the concept of suffering on behalf of humanity, but because both figures mediated between heaven and earth. Finally Prometheus was unbound by Heracles, reconciled with Zeus, and assisted him in the final battle between good and evil (Graves, 1960). The Greeks created a festival in his honor which involved carrying fire from one island to another concealed in a fennel bulb, the means by which Prometheus was postulated to have carried the fire out of

Olympus (Graves, 1960). This is perhaps the origin of today's Olympic torch relay.

Similar stories abound in many cultures. In the Irish myth, Oisin was invited into Tir na Nog (the land of eternal youth) by Naimh of the Golden Hair (Graves, 1960). On the way he slayed a giant and as a consequence Naimh was awarded to him as his wife. After 300 years (but only 3 weeks in Tir na Nog) with her as his wife, he longed for his companions and decided to return to Ireland. She gave him a white horse and told him to avoid touching any part of the earth or he would not be able to get back to her. As time passed, he became confused by the changes that he saw in Ireland. He saw some people struggling to move a huge rock and with his fairy powers hurled it away for them. Immediately, he turned into an old man and was unable to return to Tir na Nog. By a simple helpful action, one that befitted a hero, he lost his youth and his powers. Instead, as an old man representing the heroic past, he engaged in debate with St. Patrick in which he defended the pagan customs of the Fianna in the face of the new Christian austerity (Alspach, 1943; Jokinen, 2007; MacKillop, 2004). The moral of this story was that altruism was a value unto itself, worthy of sacrificing youth and all material goods for. Themes of altruism as a human good worth aspiring to can be found in many other tales, illustrating the deep rootedness of this trait in human beings and its importance (reflected in culture as well as in evolution as proposed by biologists) for the maintenance of groups to ensure their survival.

As Peterson (2000) states: "The hero's…journey from the safety of the community into the lair of the treasure-hoarding dragon, and his return bearing magical (read: 'functional') riches" is usually voluntary (p. 14). The journey constitutes a quest for ultimate meaning because it is a matter of choice (which has to be altruistic if it is to be ultimately meaningful), illustrating the importance and meaningfulness of human agency. For example, Prometheus voluntarily chose to steal the fire and bring it down to human beings. Oisin voluntarily chose to fight the giant to free the Princess of the fairies. None of these heroes was compelled to undertake the adventurous quest in search for meaning. Of course, in some cases, the hero does not choose the journey but is compelled by some authority, or perhaps a taboo or a social obligation, to undertake it. Oisin was perhaps obliged by his warrior status, as well as by love, to fulfill his quest with Niamh, but his choice whether or not to stay in Tir na Nog underpinned his desire and choice to return to his companions of his own volition.

Another example of the voluntary choice of a hero's quest can be found in the Story of The Golden Blackbird (Lang, 1892; Winther, 2004). In this story, the King was ill and a foreign doctor divined that he would die unless a golden blackbird was found. The King sent his sons out, beginning with the eldest, to find the golden blackbird. The sons had no choice but to set off on their quest for the bird. However, despite their obligations to their father they decided to abandon the journey and enjoy themselves at an inn, figuring that if their father died, it was to their advantage since they would inherit his wealth. They soon ran out of money and they were kept as prisoners against their debts. The youngest son on the other hand chose a different path and decided to commit to completing the mission of obtaining the golden blackbird and so became the hero. He could have joined his two elder brothers in a life of merriment and wait for his father to die but he chose to continue on his journey to find the bird. In the story, he found that he could only obtain the blackbird in exchange for a porcelain maiden. When he was successful, he returned to secure the release of his brothers (another voluntary heroic act). They rewarded him by trying to drown him and take the bird to their father themselves. Order was restored when the youngest son appeared and the Porcelain Maiden revealed that he was the one who had found both her and the blackbird. The two brothers were put to death.

The story clearly indicates that it is possible to submit to immediate pleasure rather than to altruistic service, but the consequences are not desirable. Greed turns the world upside down and everyone loses, once again underscoring the importance of altruism over personal pleasure and greed. Thus, communities appear to create folktales, myths and legends as part of their overall search for life meaning, which in turn emphasize the values (in this case altruism) undergirding their cultural ideals. In these tales, heroes and heroines represent what may be perceived as both the ultimate human aspiration (to engage in selfless action for the purpose of constructing and rejuvenating the world for the sake of human survival [Peterson, 2000]), and meaning of existence. Retelling the exploits of heroic mythical figures enables people to represent their quest for meaning, offering a means of identification and an ideal. As mentioned earlier, often mythical and religious figures have similar origins. The legend of Prometheus for instance seems to share some elements with the story of Jesus. Both figures heroically sacrificed themselves for the good of humanity.

While Chiriack (2007) opined that folktales represented human aspirations, the psychoanalyst Jung (1983/1953) saw them as describing the journey of individuation where the polar parts of the psyche were reconciled in order for individuals to be psychically integrated, or to understand their personal story. For example, in the Golden Blackbird story, the King (masculine principle, represented by consciousness, or what Jung referred to as the animus) needed to be reconciled with the feminine principle (what Jung called the anima), represented by the Porcelain Maiden. The anima and animus needed to be reconciled in order for wholeness to be achieved (though the Porcelain Maiden revealed the true story to the old king, she actually signified the continuation of this principle in the youngest son, who became king). In Jungian terms, the story can be interpreted as a metaphor for reclamation of the feminine principle in a society that has become increasingly masculine and lost its balance (Winther, 2004). But while this would be described by Jung as a symbolic relationship between archetypal principles pervading all society, it is also a journey that every individual has to make in his/her development as a person. Jung (1983/1953) argued that we all have to integrate our feminine and masculine, introversion and extraversion, sensing and feeling, etc. in order to attain psychic maturity or what he called integrity.

Therefore, the quest for meaning dramatized in folktales is first and foremost a psychic journey, illustrating human development.

Chinen (1990) argued that in some tales, young heroes and heroines were allowed to get away with evil deeds for which they were excused on the basis that they were under the spell of powerful villains. An example is the male Beast figure in the Beauty and the Beast who turned out to be enchanted, and was finally revealed to be an eligible young prince (LePrince de Beaumont, 1783/2009). The typical developmental task of childhood through adolescence to young adulthood was characterized in these tales by the projection of negative traits to others. Having been put under a spell by some evil force, from which they needed to be rescued, they avoided taking responsibility for their actions. As Chinen (1990) pointed out, adolescents frequently claimed that their parents, teachers, and others in authority were wicked and rebelled against them. Such projection "is often normal and helpful in youth" (Chinen, 1990, p. 22). It seemed to be part of the process of enabling the expression of individuality, but could not be continued in adult life. In the second half of life, such projection had to cease and responsibilities had to be owned. Elderly protagonists tended to be punished for evil deeds and were not allowed to project or attribute them to villainous influences. According to Chinen (1990), these tales dramatized the journey through life as played out in human moral development.

The basic point here is that folktales, myths, and legends symbolise human aspirations, psychic development and integration, or construction and rejuvenation. Apart from being a means of cultural entertainment, they are a significant means through which human beings have searched for meaning throughout history, and in every culture. Folktales, myths, legends, and their re-incarnation in artistic forms such as ballads have always been a part of everyday life, an element of folk knowledge which helps communities to sustain themselves by affirming their sense of identity, helping people to rehearse social principles and incorporate new experiences into existing traditions (Buchan, 1997; Jones 1995; Palmer, 1988; Percy, 1966). Normal daily occupations can be a very important means of empowering individuals as they strive to create narratives that symbolically resemble folktales, myths, and legends in which they are heroes, helping them to realize ultimate meaning (by enabling them to construct and rejuvenate their lives).

Intellectual inquiry and the search for meaning

The French historian Michel Bloch (cited in Depaepe, 2007, p. 28) wrote:

> What man who has grown old in his trade has never wondered, with a pang in his heart, whether he has spent his life intelligently?

Throughout history, the importance of intellectual inquiry through philosophy and science has imbued human beings with a sense of meaning. The English worker-writers whose autobiographies featured in chapter two were probably acting in accordance with earlier traditions of auto-didacticism amongst working class people. They were expressing themselves through exploration and creativity, which were intellectual endeavors. As we stated in the beginning of the chapter, this human need to search for meaning is what prompted the rise of philosophy, which probably started with the appreciation of cause and effect relationships and led to the rise of religion (Wolpert, 2007).

The development of philosophy in ancient Greece in the 6th century BC was "something wholly new and one of the most important milestones in human development" (Magee, 1998, p. 12). In this intellectual journey, human beings attempted to answer questions such as what things were made of (Thales), the meaning of opposites, and whether reality was permanent or transitory (Heraclitus, Permenides), as well as to answer moral questions such as the meaning of justice, right and wrong ways of living, etc. (Socrates) (Hergenhahn, 1997; Magee, 1998). Western philosophers attempted "to understand the world by the use of their reason, without appealing to religion, or revelation, or authority, or tradition" (Magee, 1998, p. 12), or as Russell (1961, p. 14) argued, in terms of "what we can know" rather than in terms of a theological "dogmatic belief that we have knowledge where in fact we have ignorance". The rediscovery of ancient Greek authors during the 15th century which characterized the renaissance and the emergence of humanistic thought led to the beginning of modern rational thinking as a way of understanding the world and human existence.

From the beginning, Western philosophical thinkers attempted to understand reality in a scientific manner. The search for the truth was positivistic, objective, and empirical. For example, Thales postulated (based on his observations and reasoning) that everything is made of the same substance, which he thought was water [he was correct in the assertion that there was something unique underlying all existing things, although now we know that it is pure energy rather than a "substance" such as water (Capra, 1999, 1996; Hawking, 1988)]. Plato, among others, developed sophisticated theories about biological species and a taxonomy of biological genera based on similarity of form. Of course Plato's genera were based on his teleological theory of form, in which each species developed by actualizing its potential to become what it was destined to become (Ariew, n.d.). According to Plato, "the striving towards good depends on a standard of excellence in the forms" (Ariew, n.d., p. 7). Thus, the striving towards good for a seed depends on the standard of what it is to be the best tree that the seed is destined to be. Similarly, the striving towards good for an unborn child depends on the conception of what it is to be a fine grown man or woman whom the developing fetus represents. Conceptually, in Plato's view, the meaning in life for any individual is in eventually actualizing the potential to become whoever one is destined to be.

This confluence of science and philosophy continued until the rise of empiricist thinkers in the mid-1700s, such as John Locke, George Berkley and David Hume. Such people repudiated pure reason and advocated sense experience as the most reliable source of knowledge (Hergenhahn, 1997), i.e. that what we understand about the world is based on what we can verify through our own observations. A full discussion of the history of the evolution of ideas is beyond the scope of this book, but it is important to note that at this point science became separated from philosophy through its pursuit of the empirical. Scientists focused primarily on the pursuit of knowledge by gathering sense data while philosophers persisted on attempts to arrive at the truth through reasoning and analysis of the structure of language.

Auguste Compte's empiricism in the 18th century was the culmination of positivism (Hergenhahn, 2004). Compte suggested that scientists should just gather and report pure sense data without much interpretation and synthesis, because any interpretation would be a distortion of reality. However, with the discovery of phenomena such as electromagnetism, the form of radical empiricism advocated by Compte's positivism became problematic. Phenomena such as electromagnetism, quantum mechanics, and gravity could not be observed directly by human beings using their senses, but their influence could be sensed. They had to be inferred logically from observations. This necessity for inference made pure positivism insufficient as a scientific method. Due to these difficulties, a number of German scientists who were trained in logic, mathematics, and physics met at the University of Vienna in 1907 to discuss and try to figure out a solution (McKelvey, 1997). Finally, the term "logical positivism" was coined by Herbert Fiegl as a compromise between Compte's positivism and the necessity for logical inference due to the newly discovered scientific phenomena.

It is therefore clear that the intellectual journey in pursuit of meaning has led to two consequences: 1) scientific development; and 2) increased self-knowledge which according to Socrates (and modern psychological thinking) is the basis of virtuous living (Hergenhahn, 1997; Magee, 1998). Occupational therapists are not new to the need to facilitate good living through self-knowledge. They use reflections and personal stories all the time to help foster client-centered therapy and to facilitate client growth. Both scientific development and increase in self-knowledge in this remarkable journey are highly significant to human beings. Development of science has facilitated unprecedented innovation that has been invaluable to human adaptation and survival. Similarly, the development of self-knowledge to underpin meaningful existence has been a principal resource for ideas concerning social cohesion, and maintenance of professional values through reflection.

While self-knowledge is vital to the recognition of personal meaning, it cannot be disengaged from the wider socioeconomic and political context in peoples' lives. The capacity for some individuals to own cultural capital while others lack it as discussed earlier in this chapter suggests that the question is larger than the issue of whose meaning is held to be most significant. It is also a question of who determines the means by which meaning can be explored. Definition of which meaning can be explored limits the range of questions that can be asked, data that can be gathered, and the way in which those data can be analyzed, reported, and disseminated. You or I may be aware of our experiences but what may be more important is the question of who gets to decide which experiences are relevant or useful in social life. These issues still depend on external factors, power relationships, capacities and resources. Ultimately, these relationships may determine the way in which we perceive 'objective realities'. They may also affect the resources available to us, to help us develop the questions that must first arise in ourselves in response to what we perceive.

Conclusion

The human quest for meaning has been epic in scale. Meaning has been pursued for a long time, and will continue to be pursued. In this chapter, we have attempted to find grounding of the quest for meaning in cultural traditions, religion, and creations such as myths/legends/folktales, as well as intellectual inquiry. Many of the issues discussed here ultimately stem from practical concerns, and although they may be addressed through philosophical exploration or scientific enquiry, much of the reason for their significance is because of their application in everyday life, like the gifts of Prometheus. The majority of people in the world are not engaged in scientific research or philosophical studies, but in the struggle for survival. Thus, the means of survival are the ultimate sources of meaning because they can be considered to be fundamentally existential.

Some of the findings of the study discussed in the previous chapter indicated how a cultural sense of belonging, expressed through everyday activities, is a significant source of meaning in peoples' lives. One example was how migrants to the UK often tried to fit into their host culture and ways in which people developed their own resources, and found ways to gather socially to celebrate their own cultural events and to create what De Certeau termed 'micro histories', based in their immediate surroundings (De Certeau, 1998; De Certeau et al., 1998). Wilcock (2006) emphasized the importance of doing, being, becoming and belonging, which meant that people were who they were through what they did with other people. This concept may in some ways be similar to the South African concept of 'Ubuntu', in which it is recognized that we are only human through other humans. This notion emphasizes the importance of everyday experiences that connect one to other people. Such experiences are crucial to the adaptation of human beings as members of communities, who develop cultural traditions to help them react adequately to environmental challenges.

In this chapter, we have seen that intellectual discourse is a means by which human beings adapt and find life meaning. As an example, Russell (1961) suggests that the ideas underpinning modern professional philosophies first arose from the disaffection of educated people over the venal and corrupt church and nobility who employed them. Both the monarchy and the church lost authority and people returned to the pragmatism of Greek philosophy to develop new ideas. The intellectual journey on which they embarked was shaped by the political, economic, and cultural environment of the time, and therefore was an attempt by these people to adapt to their circumstances. That is what made those intellectual pursuits so meaningful. Using intellectual reasoning to adapt was evident in the pragmatic compromises that thinkers often found that they had to make based on the reality of the time. For example, Russell (1961) pointed out that some of the new humanists recognized that despite their employers' corruption, they still had to work for them in order to have access to the materials which enabled them to pursue their intellectual activities.

It is imperative that professionals and scholars who specialize in trying to understand the meaning of human occupations (occupational therapists and occupational scientists) understand this search for meaning using multiple vehicles so that they can effectively guide and enable people to understand how what they do in their every-day occupations fits into this journey. The purpose of this book is to achieve that objective by helping individuals think about how what they do in their daily lives fits into their individual journeys in search for meaning, so that they can make choices and act in such a way that their lives are optimally meaningful. We will explore some of these narratives of meaning in another chapter.

Apply the ideas discussed in chapter 3

Exploring ways of optimizing/enriching the search for meaning in life through daily occupations in the context of cultural, religious, and intellectual institutions

After reading this chapter, help your client to explore the ways in which her journey towards attaining/enhancing meaning can be optimized. As we have discussed, throughout history, the search for meaning by humanity has constituted a journey. The symbolic vehicles used in this journey include adherence to cultural traditions, religious affiliations and practices, mythical/ legendary/fairytale narratives, and intellectual inquiry. Now, ask your client to take a moment to think and reflect, and answer the following questions as accurately and exhaustively as possible:

1. **What vehicles are your client using in the quest for meaning in life?**

a. Adherence to cultural traditions
b. Religious practice
c. Transcendence to magical reality through imaginative narratives
d. Creation of a narrative of her own hero's journey through what she does every day.
e. Intellectual pursuits

As all these vehicles are abstract, assist your client to visualize them as actual vehicles. For example, she may visualize her vehicle(s) as: a favorite animal that she can ride; the steam train of cultural tradition; the bicycle of intellectual pursuits; the barque of transcendence to magical reality; the warhorse of religious practice; a Matatu on the highway to enlightenment; and so on. Ask the client to create her own vehicles. If the client is artistically endowed, she can draw the vehicles. She can also describe them in any way that is appropriate for the individual (for example, the client can paint a picture of the vehicles in words, in poetry, etc.). The client can imagine riding the vehicles and enjoying the ride.

This activity may enable the client to visualize the next part of the exercise which is as follows:

2. Ask him to explain what the personal quest for meaning feels like;

a. What does the journey look/feel like?
b. Where is he in this journey?
c. Who/what are the people or things that are important to the client as he embarks on the journey?

Again, in thinking about this journey it may help if the client visualizes it in some metaphorical sense. For example, if the hero's narrative is written from the top of a camel the client may feel a little seasick. The camel need not, of course be in a desert. He could be riding it to the mall or in the slow lane of the freeway.

3. What can your client do to enrich the quest for meaning?

Have him continue to think about this metaphorically. For example, the journey could be conceptualized as a visit to a country of learning. Perhaps, in the journey, the client wants to stop in some places and explore them rather than just passing by, or there are experiences that he could try, such as tasting foods, hiking to explore the terrain, etc. as he continues on the journey. Perhaps the client could prepare for the journey before embarking on it by reading a guidebook of the country, learning the language of the citizens of the country, etc.

Chapter 4
Specific sources of meaning in people's lives

Learning Objectives

By the end of this chapter, the reader will demonstrate understanding of:

1. How relationships, work/leisure activities, and commitment to religious, philosophical, and/or political idea systems are used by people as sources of meaning
2. Three dimensions of meaning (having a purpose in life, having a sense of control in one's life, and being able to express one's values) and how they are experienced by people in their lives
3. How to help clients reflect about the major sources of meaning in their lives
4. The dimensions of meaning that clients experience as they arise out of the sources of meaning identified in number one above

Contents of this chapter

- Search for meaning as a never ending quest
- Sources that invest occupations with meaning
    - o Emotionally intense relationships with others
    - o Work and leisure activities, and
    - o Conviction and commitment to idea systems

- Dimensions of meaning that can be accessed through occupations
    - o Self-worth
    - o Sense of purpose
    - o Sense of control
    - o Sense of values

Introduction

In the last chapter we examined the vehicles that human beings use in their journey in search for meaning. Now the question is 'what are the wells from which they draw what they need in order to quench their thirst for that meaning on this perennial journey?' The quest for meaning is generally understood to be never ending until one ceases to exist in this life. However, there are points at which meaning is sufficiently understandable to be recognized as such, or else people would have nothing by which to make sense of the coherence of their experience. A perception of meaning may be developed from many incidents and events over the course of life, but these are ordered to shape the interpretation, rather than being understood chronologically. A useful concept that might help us understand the perception of meaning in life might be the notion of narrative time. As Mattingly (1998) and Ricouer (1980) explained, time is not linear in a narrative. It can move back and forth in order for the reader to make sense of the story. As readers, or as people compiling the story from experiences, we can witness simultaneous events and place them side by side, or move forward and backward between events in the narrative so that we can place these experiences in the meaningful context of a chain of events. The true significance of an event might be immediate, or it might be revealed later when other events have also taken place to bring about further experience, rather like a line of dominoes.

The narrator and the reader can move the vantage point by juxtaposing different events - even events happening at different times (as in the movie *The Hours*) or flipping back the pages to re-read passages that may not have been correctly understood. The pace of events can also be at variance within the same story. Thus, in the Irish myth of Oisin and Naimh presented in chapter three, the time in Tir na Nog is short. When Oisin returns to Ireland, he quickly becomes an old man, and finds that his relatives are dead. This characteristic of narrative time allows the meaning itself to change. So, in terms of the affiliations and relationships, a relationship which may have felt intense may in time cease to be so. A political affiliation developed in youth may seem redundant at a later stage in life, and yet at still further stages those events, relationships, and affiliations can be reassessed as significant. This might explain why occasionally people marry their childhood sweethearts after many years of living with others and having families with them. External factors also play a large part in determining whether events are perceived as significant. In the video *Did you know* (Fisch, 2008), possible effects of technological changes on society were explored, in which predictions were made that in future, people will hold many different jobs over their lifetimes because of these transitions. The movie exaggerates many issues, but Nick (the second author) can verify some of the predictions. He trained as a radio journalist using large reel to reel tape recorders, but now the industry uses digital recording, while mobile phones and laptops are frequently used directly as reporting devices. Even listeners can use these devices to send in their own reports. He was also a bus conductor using a hand cranked machine to issue tickets, but now ticket issuing is done by the driver and is often digitalised. Some passenger transport systems are ticketless. These occupations and their underlying meanings have changed and will continue to change over time.

From this discussion, we can surmise that maybe the search for meaning never ends and therefore one never arrives at the destination. Instead, there could be oases of meaning all along the never ending journey. So, the question is: what is the nature of that spring that becomes the source of meaning at a particular instance for the individual in his/her life journey? Since we argued in chapter three that individuals use culture, religion, folktales, intellectual pursuits, and the associated everyday activities as vehicles to carry them in their journey in search for meaning, once they arrive at their destination, or come across what they are looking for along the way, how do they know or understand that meaning?

One may argue that paradoxically, the very vehicles that convey people in their quest for meaning are also the wellsprings of meaning for which they are searching. Thus, as discovered in the analysis of the English worker-writer autobiographies in chapter two, it can be argued that the sources of meaning for many people include cultural and religious affiliations, engagement in activities that help them transcend their mundane lives, those that make them exercise their intellectual abilities thus making them feel creative, or simply those which enable them to express their identities, to be who they are. These sources of meaning were identified by Frankl (1997, 1985) and summarized quite effectively by McNamee (2007) as follows:

1. Emotionally intense relationships with others
2. Work and leisure activities, and
3. Conviction and commitment to idea systems. (p. 3 of 15)

Furthermore, according to Hughes (2006), meaning may be conceptualized as comprising of four dimensions:

Self-worth

This is crucial for establishment of relationships which are very important sources of meaning. People who have high levels of self-esteem also tend to be more socially integrated making their lives more meaningful.

Purpose

Having a purpose in life creates a feeling of connectedness with other people, because self-transcending purpose is often altruistic and therefore focusses on benefiting others other than oneself

Sense of control

This refers to the feeling that one is capable (also known as a sense of efficacy). Efficacy makes achievement of goals and therefore one's purpose in life possible. Efficacy also alludes to a sense of competency or mastery, which as we mentioned in chapter 2, is a significant source of meaning in life.

Values

These facilitate prioritization and justification of choices and subsequent actions. Without some kind of valuation system, action and achievement of goals and one's purpose in life are not possible.

In some situations people are detrimentally affected (experience poor health and may even die) if the above outlined dimensions of meaning are absent in their experiences. Bettleheim (1970), who like Frankl was a survivor of the Nazi concentration camps, narrated how his fellow inmates were systematically deprived by the guards of the means to see their continued existence as meaningful by depriving them of a sense of self-worth, purpose, choice and control, and opportunity to act in accordance with their personal values. As a result, some inmates simply gave up the will to live. He reported that he survived by deciding to do a psychological study based on his own experiences. Frankl (1997), who had already been working as a doctor in a Vienna ghetto (Pytell, 2007) found ways to treat people in order to help them manage the trauma they were experiencing in the concentration camp conditions.

Both Frankl and Bettelheim wrote about their experiences and developed psychological theories based on those experiences which have been significant contributions to the understanding of survival. Both also survived because they imbued their lives with meaning through these studies, which gave them a purpose for surviving, increased their sense of self-worth, increased their sense of control in their circumstances, and helped them articulate values that made their lives worth living. One criticism of these works has been that they arose from "a moderate form of extreme experience in concentration camps" (Pytell, 2007, p. 645). Pytell (2007) and Adamczyk (2005) contrast Frankl's and Bettelheim's experiences with those of other survivors and conclude that the uplifting impression of hope Frankl described was probably unusual. Pytell's view was that Frankl's and Bettelheim's accounts perhaps deal more with their psychological processing of the experiences they underwent than constituting a generalizable theory.

It is important to note that both Frankl (1985) and Bettelheim (1970) described in some detail the controversial phenomenon of 'Moslems' or 'Musselmänner', people who gave up on their ability to survive, describing it as a major cause of death. In addition, Frankl worked under the auspices of the Nazi controlled Rothschild hospital injecting and applying drugs directly into the brains of Jewish suicide victims (Pytell, 2007, 2000). In Frankl's (1985) therapeutic system of 'logotherapy' and in his other texts (for example, Frankl, 1978, 1969) he cited himself and his colleagues' use of paradoxical intention as a miracle cure. Pytell (2007, p. 656) described use of paradoxical intention as "insensitivity", and asserted that Frankl's religious overtones often belied the true complexities of many clients' circumstances. These criticisms not-withstanding, it cannot be denied that both Frankl and Bettelheim found meaning in their intellectualization of the concentration camp experiences which made the terrible and perhaps absurd comprehensible to them. This ability to find meaning in dire circumstances through articulation and interpretation of experiences into a comprehensible intellectual system probably contributed to their own survival.

Activity that helps one express personal agency provides purpose and therefore meaning in difficult circumstances. Davies (1991) described how many people in prisons turn to writing, partly because some form of writing materials can be obtained and spirited into the cells relatively easily, but also because the activity of writing makes reflection possible and provides a sense of control in an enclosed space which affords a paucity of meaningful activities in which to engage and in which one's life otherwise feels out of control. wa Thiong'o (1982) for example wrote his book *Detained: A prisoner's diary* while in detention, in defiance of authorities that had plucked him out of professorial heights and thrown him in the dungeon of a maximum security prison because of his expression of disapproval of the excesses of government. By writing the book on pieces of toilet paper and smuggling it out to the publishers, he felt a sense of triumph over the authorities because he was still able to exercise control of his thought processes and to communicate his criticism of authority to others outside the prison walls despite all attempts to silence him.

There is a considerable body of prison writing in all kinds of genres spanning many centuries. Much of it is about the very basic necessities such as food, sleep, and other essentials that are denied prisoners, making their very survival a challenge – see, for example the semi-autobiographical novels of Victor Serge, such as *The Case of Comrade Tulayev* (Serge, 1968/1948). Obviously, being reduced to a struggle for the basic necessities for survival is demeaning and life changing.

Pytell's attempt to discredit Frankl's and Bettelheim's experiences as a "moderate form of extreme experience" belies the issue that for each of us, unfortunate or catastrophic events can take us to places in which we have not been before and unlike anything else that we have previously undergone. We do not have the knowledge of previous experiences on which to draw in order to understand how to react, even though we may know other people who have encountered something similar. Examples of common events that cause people considerable anxiety and grief include the death of a loved one, a severe illness, disability, or the likelihood of spending some time in a psychiatric facility. It's not a question of whether such experiences are more or less severe than others; they present situations where individuals, and possibly their relatives are not able to control the things that are happening to them. In those circumstances, events can be frightening, and fundamentally disempowering. As one of the second authors' psychiatric clients once stated, "mental illness is not like breaking a leg, in which case in about three months you'll be about walking; you never know whether you're going to be ill again, or how bad it will get." Consequently it would be unfair to dismiss Frankl's and Bettelheim's experiences as not being useful representations of the trials and tribulations of concentration camp experiences. They were real enough.

Consistent with the dimension of meaning related to a feeling of being in control, loss of capacity to do things for oneself presents one with great fear. Frankl (1978, 1969) gave a number of examples of people who perceived themselves as having lost a sense of purpose in life following severe injury and becoming disabled making them feel incapable of doing things for themselves and therefore making them feel a sense of loss of control in their lives. This feeling of loss of control was confounded by the inability to enjoy every aspect of their lives. People with experiences of disability are often subject to multiple exclusions which are rooted in social attitudes. Mason (2002) and Neville-Jan (2004) describe the difficulties they had as persons with disabilities in being able to fulfill the demands of their roles as mothers. People with disabilities frequently find that their relationships, sexual intimacy and expression and other areas of human social life are made difficult to negotiate by *ablist* social pressures (Abbot, 2012). That is why Whiteford (2000, 1997) was prompted to develop the term occupational deprivation to describe these situations where people are denied opportunities to participate in typical meaningful activities. Such deprivation leads to a decreased sense of meaning in life. In this chapter Hughes' dimensions of meaning will be discussed further, and their connection to the quest for meaning as discussed in chapter 3 will be explored.

Sources of meaning

Despite the caveats concerning his past, Frankl was at the forefront of the intellectual discourse and therapeutic focus on issues pertaining to meaning in the 20th century. The extremes of the Nazi oppression created many intensely difficult situations for those concentration camp victims who were able to survive. Whether Frankl developed his theories contemporaneously with these experiences or, as Pytell (2007, 2003, 2000) contended, in retrospect, these theories have been widely disseminated and have been very influential in the world of psychotherapy. For Frankl (1997), meaning resulted from the ability to: be creative in whatever one did; love another person or thing; and hope for the future. A key element in the expression of humanness, Frankl (1992, 1966) wrote, was self-transcendence. This term describes a specific quality of people who are able to look beyond personal needs, wants, desires, and even tribulations, and are able to pursue the objective of being part of something that is bigger than them, and of loving and serving other people or greater causes. Such people establish connectedness with the world around them.

Frankl contrasted the principle of transcendence with other psychological approaches focusing on the maintenance of individual stability or satisfaction. In his view, personal equilibrium is not so much a function of internal stability but the ability to relate to other people. Frankl (1969) described individuals as being comparable to pieces in a mosaic. A community is composed of individuals and like a mosaic, needs all the individuals in order for the overall picture to be clear. This is to say that the patterns consisting of responsibilities and obligations, and the meaning of individual lives, are all expressed through the fulfillment or meeting of shared values in a community. In this conceptualization, the community depends on individuals, and individuals require a community.

Since Frankl, other scholars have further investigated and discussed these postulated sources of meaning. In one study, Thompson (1993) found that older adults found meaning in work, leisure activities, grand-parenting, and intimacy (having close relationships that were mutually nurturing). He found that relationships (the theme of connectedness to other human beings discussed in chapter two) were a central component of all the other sources of meaning. It is instructive that relationships were identified by Frankl as a significant source of meaning in peoples' lives. Paul, Miller, and Paul (1997) argued that "the activities that give meaning to one's life will give one reasons for acting that are, to some extent, independent of self-interest – reasons derived from the worth of the activities themselves" (p. xii). In this statement, Paul et al. seemed to suggest that meaning came out of engagement in activities that were deemed worthwhile unto themselves. They seemed to agree with Frankl (1992) that such activities often derived their value from being performed for the benefit of something or someone other than one-self, or for the purpose of experiencing and loving another person as a unique being.

This is a continuation of the notion of self-transcendence offered by Frankl as a significant source of meaning as discussed earlier. It is also an extension of the idea of the existential importance of the principle of altruism discussed in chapter three. Doing things for the benefit of others is acknowledged by economists and political philosophers such as Smith (1999), Keynes (1936/2003) and others as a way of preserving social stability to enable distribution of goods. Even pirate societies recognized the importance of altruism (Exquemelin, 1678/1969), and developed a system of welfare that offered benefits and property sharing. Leading thinkers in modern times are beginning to make arguments for the need to return to a focus on this altruistic concern for the greater good, for the sake of our world and the human family. For example, Max-Neef (1991) generated a list of human values which are determinants of a form of prosperity that is not expressed in monetary terms, but in access to leisure, space for intimacy, friendships, and other ways of meeting human needs that do not focus entirely on self-interest.

The primacy of relationships to meaning in life goes counter to the thinking among many people (Calvinist Protestants, Chinese, the Ancient Greeks, and Romans for example) that what gives a person's life meaning is hard work, wise use of time, and acquisition of wealth. However, Bruni (2006) suggests that material wealth is a source of meaning only in so far as it elicits the admiration of the owner by other people; admiration by others becomes the true source of meaning and wealth or the appearance of wealth is just a means to that end. James (2006) described how English middle class people attached great importance to appearances. For example, they would use net curtains in their front windows to obscure the furniture and effects in the rooms inside; socially superior neighbours occasionally sneered at items they thought to be merely aspirational, while socially inferior neighbours would be tempted to steal objects they found desirable. This attribution of the source of meaning may contradict arguments that meaning cannot be found from without (such as being given accolades by others), but rather from within oneself. For those who subscribe to this view, the problem of meaninglessness that Frankl (1997, 1969) talked about may be attributed precisely to the social emphasis on the external at the expense of the internal sources of meaning. None the less, as Allan (1989) and Thompson (1993) found in their studies, social relationships presented important and complex sources of meaning for many people, as will be discussed later.

Cultural and religious affiliation

In chapter three, we discussed how the formation of social groups was a means of evolutionary adaptation that helped human beings survive. This notion was supported in current literature where affiliation to groups was clearly identified as a source of meaning for many people. Like Frankl, Haidt (2006) argued that the relationship to self, others, work, and a higher power were important sources of happiness (and therefore meaning, assuming that happy people consider their lives meaningful at the moment of happiness). This perspective mirrored that by Putman (1995) who argued that social relationships were forms of capital that people used to advance their well-being, including economic health (for example by enhancing job attainment and investment opportunities through such networks). He argued that the traditional forms of social capital maintained through these relationships were in decline in the USA (and perhaps in other parts of the world as well).

Putnam explained how people had come to invest their social capital in their work communities at the expense of the communities they lived in, because work and living communities became separated as sites of human activity. Communities became increasingly fragmented by the arrival of television, which encouraged people to stay at home and engage passively as an audience rather than participating actively in communal pastimes. This erosion of social capital has many consequences, such as the replacement of close relationships with amenities. For example high street businesses and shops such as the local baker or the butcher that De Certeau et al. (1998) described have been replaced by the ubiquitous supermarket and the mall which are convenient but ultimately facilitate anonymity. These developments represent some of the larger global macroeconomic forces, indicated by high street brands, the internet, and other mass social elements which change peoples' habits. It would be wrong to cast these issues as simply good or bad (Stolle & Hooghe, 2004). For example new forms of participation, such as internet based social networking through the computer are a significant means of connection for many people across generations (Kaplan & Haenlein, 2010). These networks also offer many positive opportunities for development of lasting friendships and learning about people from other cultures in an international arena where fellow players may often come from other countries.

In regard to Haidt's (2006), Thompson's (1993), and Frankl's (1969) assertion that the source of meaning for many people is relationship to self, other people, and a higher being, as Haidt (2006) states, this is so because human beings are made for love, relationships, and family, and without those things, they cannot find happiness. Haidt (2006) further argues that the lives of human beings only make sense within the context of membership to a higher entity, such as a religious organization, school of thought, scientific or political organization. The necessity for membership to a larger entity is consistent with Putman's (1995, 2000) notion of social capital and the earlier discussion of the evolutionary importance of altruism. Furthermore, to make full sense of a person's life, the organization to which she belongs should have a noble purpose and be grounded on a long past consisting of established traditions (this alludes to the importance of culture as a source of meaning, but sometimes the meaning is also derived from distancing oneself from long-held cultural traditions that one may judge to be unethical or against human good, such as slavery or oppression of women).

In this sense, traditional heritage informs the present while shaping the future. This is best articulated by the Jewish Reconstructionists (Jewish Reconstructionist Federation, 2013), who consider Judaism to be a dynamic and continuously evolving faith which necessitates dealing with doubts and questions in order to determine life meaning. Their website offers the following statement:

> We believe 'the past has a vote.' Therefore we struggle to hear the voices of our ancestors and listen to their claim on us (read through traditions they pass down through generations) ...

They continue to illustrate how these traditions inform and give meaning to their life choices by guiding them in posing questions such as: "What might this custom or that idea mean to us today? What might we borrow from the custom to create a new tradition that is more significant for us today?" (p. 2 of 5). Further, Congar (2004) points to the importance of cultural traditional values as a source of meaning because they provide a sense of identity and continuity. This notion seems to be consistent with Tevye's (Jewison, 1971) statement in the movie *Fiddler on the roof* that traditions provide stability to a community. According to Congar (2004), if you are walking on a road, one foot has to be on the ground while the other is off the ground. This condition allows meaningful movement forward. You cannot make progress if both feet are continuously planted on the ground. However, you cannot keep both feet off the ground simultaneously either.

To give a personal example, the first author comes from the Meru people of Kenya. Among the Meru, one tradition that is revered and continues to be practiced without fail is initiation (through circumcision) of males as a way of transitioning them from boyhood to manhood. Part of this initiation includes intense education about the ways of the Meru people, how to be respectful to parents and especially to the mother and the womenfolk in general, how to behave appropriately and not to shame oneself or one's family or the community, etc. Continuation of this tradition ensures that Meru men remain grounded in values that provide them with identity by connecting them to a larger group of people from the past to the present (the Meru ancestry), providing them with a sense of value, pride, and belonging. However, while preserving such valuable traditions, the Meru people have also embraced modernity, especially Western education, technology (such as cars, modern houses, computers, and telephones). In other words, for Meru people, one foot remains grounded in cultural traditional values (such as initiation to manhood) while the other foot is up in the air as the community leaps forward into the future of modernity and technology.

Religious and other cultural traditions make it possible to stay grounded while at the same time we make progress and adapt through experiences that we gain in our journey through life. Perhaps that is why so many people find meaning in those traditions despite environmental, economic and social change. However, although traditions tend to be regarded as fixed, most traditional artifacts of culture are subject to change as people continue to adapt. Some values and practices may survive from one generation to the next, but others may change, and new ones may be added. Many traditions provide "continuity with a suitable historic past" (Hobsbawm, 1983, p. 1) and are used as vessels to propagate a set of established values, such as patriotism, in the public consciousness. Hobsbawm points out that even when the values of a society are disrupted by rapid changes as occurs in revolutions, those initiating the change (revolutionaries) justify their actions using historical information. Countryman (1986) indicated how this was the case for various groups of people who took part in the American Revolution that led to the creation of a new nation. Yet traditions themselves are often invented to suit the need for meaning. Hibbert's (2001) biography of Queen Victoria details how, although she was a queen associated with many English traditions, in many respects she recognised a need to break with previous values; Cannadine (1983) explores how many of the British monarchical 'traditions' were developed during the latter part of her reign or in modern times.

Some of the enduring festivities in which people take part involve less pomp and act as some kind of safety valve, allowing a certain element of mockery of social institutions. Carnivals for example allow people to make fun of different aspects of their society or to suspend certain social rules for a specified period of time. Everyone understands that such events are not a real challenge to the status quo. Other traditions may be celebrated by migrant communities in order to express communal solidarity and to share their identity with the host country. For example many Mexicans hold traditional festivities for Our Lady of Guadalupe in the US around December 12th. Many migrant households also continue to maintain little islands of culture through their décor and the meals shared by family members (Lyons & Tarrier, 2004). All these cultural festivities provide people with a means of connecting to a larger cultural entity, and that is their true meaning in peoples' lives.

Relationships

Affiliation to religious and cultural institutions and adherence to traditions provides opportunities to form relationships. People generally try to find other people with whom they have something in common, with whom they anticipate the likelihood of sharing interests and values, so that they can form groups with them. The extent to which one person is interested in another may have empathic or altruistic components, but also contains an element of reward or reciprocal feeling. Friendships arise from the kind of exchanges (gifts, compliments, support, recognition, task sharing) that are negotiated as relationships develop (Allan, 1989). Relationships, whether of love for another person (Frankl, 1985) or 'intimacy' (Thompson 1993), are significant as sources of meaning (see discussion in the beginning of this chapter). For relationships to be optimal sources of meaning however, Frankl (1969) was careful to point out that the happiness they provide should derive from a spiritual dimension directed towards the unique essence of a person, not mere human erotic infatuation. In this sense, the ultimate intimate connection to another human being through a shared sexual relationship is a means by which spiritual love can be mutually expressed.

Findings from research studies have confirmed both the spiritual essence and primacy of relationships as sources of meaning in people's lives. According to Jim and Andersen (2007, p. 366), "social interaction is associated with greater meaning: quality of family relationships are associated with increased purpose in life and religious and existential well-being". Yet the importance of other people with whom a person is able to express forms of mutuality in order to experience 'meaning' becomes a problem in a couples-oriented society (Allan, 1989). Social opportunities for single people are limited and it seems that the only way around this is to form a recognized relationship with another person, otherwise the individual may end up being isolated (Allan, 1989). When people are lonely and isolated, they may feel unhappy and disconnected, and their lives may be experienced as meaningless. The death of a loved one or disruption of an intimate relationship through desertion or divorce can lead to an extended crisis in a person's life as he/she seeks to re-establish a basis for relating socially to other people. If a couple has tended to form their friendships outside their partnership, this may be less of a problem than if their social relations revolved around them only as a couple.

Relationships facilitate a sense of belonging, which is existentially very important for human beings. In a study by Dwyer, Nordenfelt and Ternestedt (2008), nursing home residents informed the researchers how valuable their familial relationships were in providing them with "a sense of belonging and having communication and relationships with others" (p. 100). Much of the significance of relationships derives from what Frankl (1966, 1997) called self-transcendence. In one program designed to treat war veterans with Post Traumatic

Stress Disorders (PTSD), the emphasis to the clients was on moving beyond the self and doing things for others or to "discover meaning through service to others, through creative endeavors, and through (re)discovering activities that offer enjoyment and personal fulfillment" (Southwick, Gilmartin, McDonough, & Morrissey, 2006, p. 166). It is also important for some people to be able to tell their story to someone else and to have their experiences believed, which can happen through the interactions afforded in community engagement.

Work and leisure occupations

According to Frankl (1997, 1985, 1966), a fundamental element of life's meaning can be found in what one does. In occupational therapy and occupational science, this can be understood as taking part in daily occupations including activities for self-care, productivity (work), and relaxation (leisure). The occupations that provide the most meaning in peoples' lives are generally those that are age appropriate and are socially recognized and meet cultural expectations (American Occupational Therapy Association [AOTA], 2002; Christiansen, 1994; Law, Polatajko, Baptiste, & Townsend, 2002). There are many reasons why engagement in occupations is significant. Occupational performance provides people with opportunities to experience a sense of: connection with others through relationships; being capable (efficacious) and therefore in control of their lives; ability to achieve important goals (Hughes, 2006); and creativity.

The view that occupations, including leisure, that are most meaningful to individuals are those that enhance a person's sense of empowerment, self-determination, and efficacy (Kelly & Kelly, 1994; Shannon & Bourque, 2005) is not new. Many years ago, Aristotle (cited in Maynard & Kleiber, 2005) described lack of a sense of efficacy as a negation of the ability to actualize one's potentiality. According to him, the value of occupations such as leisure pursuits was in their ability to enable an individual to make progress in his "quest for excellence" (p. 476). This ability to realize actuality (realness) is what, according to Aristotle, made "us uniquely human" (p. 478).

Modern societies, particularly those in which people have inherited a strong work ethic place a particular emphasis on work and productivity, which has often been reduced to the concept of having the means of supporting oneself financially. Other tasks, such as housework or caring for others without formal reimbursement, are also significant contributions to economic functioning since these are necessary parts of the process of maintaining a stable social fabric. However, such tasks are not recognized by the economic systems through financial remuneration. Emphasis on paid work as a source of meaning is troublesome considering that the industrial society has never enjoyed long periods of stability and there are often difficult economic times when opportunities for work are limited. Even during periods of relative prosperity many people can be out of work. Over the first decade of the century a more or less constant 2.7 million working age people were on welfare in the UK due to disability and long term unemployment (Brown, Hanlon, Turok, et al., 2008).

Furthermore, working purely for money can become an end in itself, producing material benefits but preventing a person from experiencing work as an important source of meaning in life. On the other hand, a period of unemployment can produce a feeling of emptiness and apathy, with the life of the jobless person appearing as if it has no meaning because he is unable to find recognized forms of work. The person may still occupy significant but unpaid voluntary and domestic or caring roles. If the person's access to social institutions is limited, this barrier may produce a detrimental effect on health and wellbeing (Paul, Geithner & Moser, 2009).

Another way in which work affects meaning in life is by making a person's occupational life grossly unbalanced. In recent years, one of the effects of long working hours in many Western cultures has been an emergence of higher rates of stress and anxiety among the working class and professional people (Briar 2006; Duxbury, Lyons & Higgins, 2008; Etherington, Lewis & Mark, 2008). Frankl (1969) and Illich (1980) point out that both individuals and communities require a balanced approach to work and leisure. They also state that some work that produces community value (such as volunteering, or being a political activist) need not produce direct economic benefits but can still provide a sense of worth for an individual and benefit the community immensely.

In considering the role of work in providing meaning in peoples' lives, changes in productive activities and how society assigns value to those activities have to be taken into consideration. For example, one important change in many Western societies has been in the nature of work. As an illustration, mining and steel industries in the US and UK have been on the decline leading to a decrease in industrial work in which many males were traditionally employed. These types of employment have been replaced by more transitory service work with more flexible hours that favor women. However, such work is not as well paying and frequently women have to take more than one job in order to meet financial needs of the family, while men are often unable to find suitable work (Grimshaw et al., 2008).

Also, individual agency (ability to make choices and act on those choices) afforded by work is fundamental to the experience of work itself as a source of meaning. The most meaningful work, according to Kelly and Kelly (1994), is that which offers a chance for self-direction through the exercise of initiative and independent judgment, and which offers an opportunity for learning new skills. More recently, authors have tried to create formulas for happiness at work. According to Kreamer (2013), many of those formulas are based on the idea that the "good life happiness" at work (p. 1 of 5) is achieved by engaging in work tasks that: are meaningful and challenging; create peak experiences (as occurs in the rare experiences of special creativity or breakthroughs at work); and provide a chance to work with a talented team of colleagues who share some larger organizational vision and a commitment to make that vision come true. The availability of such work in contemporary times is not always assured, which makes the assumption that work is always a source of meaning tenable.

While examining how what people do provides them with a sense of meaning in their lives, it is important to point out that people do not seek meaningfulness as a goal in itself. Meaning is largely context-based and therefore, as found in the worker-writers' autobiographies discussed in chapter two, it arises from the matrix of everyday practices of maintaining reciprocal relationships and engaging in mutually desired activities and events in peoples' contexts. This emergent nature of meaning is evident in the work of Frankl (1966) who distinguishes himself from his psychologist and psychoanalytic predecessors by making it clear that meaning is not gained so much from an intentional seeking of pleasure, but is a by-product of activity. This is an important difference which is sometimes missed in setting occupational goals which are often perhaps based on Maslow's individual-focused concept of self-actualization. Frankl pointed out that self-actualization is an effect of the experience of meaning, and that ultimately the meaning of a life can only be recognized once it has been lived. In his view, rather than pleasure-seeking for its own sake, people should seek experiences that produce pleasure.

None the less, the ability to engage in desired occupations has been repeatedly demonstrated to be an important source of meaning in peoples' lives. In the study by Dwyer, Nordenfelt and Ternestedt (2008) cited earlier, one of the sources of meaning for study participants was the ability to engage in enjoyable things, including simple occupations such as being able to turn on the television set or radio when one desired to do so. Similarly, a client whom the second author once worked with said that one of the things he most enjoyed about leaving the mental health ward in a psychiatric institution and staying in a home environment was being able to watch an episode of *Hawaii 5-0*. He could see the whole programme without someone else changing the channel or interrupting him. In other words, lack of occupational choice may be seen as the ultimate experience of lack of efficacy which invalidates an individual's very existence. Dwyer, Nordenfelt and Ternestedt's research participants and Nick's client found themselves to be dependent on others in every situation of their lives. This dependence on other people reduced their ability to make choices and decreased their sense of meaning in life.

In addition, Thompson (1993) found that some of the sources of meaning for older adults included participating in work and leisure activities. Work was found to be such a fundamental part of his study participants' identities that when they retired, they had difficult disengaging from it. They tried to maintain work habits in retirement. Some would perform work-like activities such as constructing home extensions; others would wake up at 5:00 am every day as they did during their working life and try to maintain the work related routines. In other studies, it has been found that unplanned retirement is a major contributor to the depression that follows unemployment (Villamil, Huppert, & Melzer, 2006). In response to the anxieties of unplanned retirement, some people try to maintain the façade of still being in the workforce. In part, this reaction is related to the stigma associated with 'not working', making some people feel the need to maintain 'work' appearances (Goffman, 1978).

This transitional problem has long been recognized in contemporary society as indicated by establishment of pre-retirement education and planning programs (Donahue, 1951; Blakely & Reibiero, 2008). Such programs usually include advising people who are about to retire on ways of developing hobbies and activities to sustain their interests post-retirement. This approach is predicated on the research findings indicating that people who remain active longer appear to enjoy longer life expectancy. As a consequence there has been a demand for pre-retirement education to help people remain engaged so as to maintain their physical and mental health (Blakely & Reibiero, 2008). However, it is not clear whether retirement is experienced in the same way by all individuals. Some people continue to participate in activities in which they were involved before retirement, while others do not experience an increase in activities after retirement as they had expected. Factors such as the degree to which retirees were involved in their previous work may determine whether or not they are able to maintain a rewarding occupational life after retirement. Gee and Braille (1999) suggested that pre-retirement education needs to go beyond the obvious and stereotypical perspectives about healthy retirement and focus on whether people are able to make the choices they need in order to have a positive experience post-retirement.

Finally, as mentioned earlier, Thompson (1993) found that leisure was another important source of meaning for older adults. Leisure refers to those occupations in which people engage purely for enjoyment [AOTA (2009), Law et al. (2002)]. The concept of leisure, as we have already mentioned, may not be shared by people in all societies, and even as a Western concept, not until recently did it become known in some communities. Thompson found that leisure activities were extremely important sources of meaning for older adults who had retired from paid work. The importance of leisure as a source of meaning has also been underscored by Shannon and Bourque (2005) who found that clients with breast cancer found enjoyable occupations to be important because they were a means of developing skills and knowledge, and therefore helping them experience a sense of self-determination, efficacy, and self-empowerment in spite of their condition. Handy (2002) argued that leisure occupations such as home maintenance, volunteering, and study (intellectual pursuits) were often perceived by individuals to be much more meaningful than paid work. As an example, he cited the experience of one woman who earned a living by packing eggs. She felt that writing television plays (which she did as a hobby) was really her work. This activity was more meaningful to her than packing eggs.

Also, because home life can include many demands which contribute to stress and anxiety, it may be difficult to separate the health effects of working conditions from those of other variables such as family life (Duxbury, Lyons, & Higgins, 2008). The quality of home life can be affected by economic and social factors such as unemployment or retirement. Ultimately, as Thompson (1993) pointed out, it is important to realize that occupations are not divorced from human relationships. In many cases, people find even more meaning in occupations that enhance the formation and maintenance of interpersonal relationships than in those occupations for which they are paid money. As Illich (1980) suggested in his concept of 'useful unemployment', many of the things that people do for each other produce social benefits without necessarily resulting in any monetary value, an observation that was made earlier in this chapter. This was consistent with Thompson's finding that his research participants valued work that provided a context in which important relationships were established. Deep friendships that develop at the work place, including romantic (intimate) ones, often last for lifetimes. Shannon and Bourque (2005) also found that the relationships that women diagnosed with breast cancer established at work were an important source of support for them.

Similarly, the most valued leisure occupations are those that are performed with other individuals and therefore help to enhance and maintain relationships. Thompson (1993) found that mutually nurturing relationships were enhanced by people doing enjoyable things, such as dancing and taking walks together. Shannon and Bourque (2005, p. 80) also found that for women with breast cancer, "spending time with friends by going to a movie, going out for coffee, visiting, or shopping" were activities they used to elicit support from friends and therefore were very significant to them. Similarly, Kelly and Kelly (1994, p. 3 of 15) pointed out that "Family and leisure are closely related in both associations and meanings". Several authors have confirmed this proposition through the auto-ethnographic investigation of how families use occupations to deal with events such as loss or childbirth, experience of disability and pain (Neville-Jan, 2004; Hoppes, 2005a, 2005b; Salmon, 2006). Neville-Jan (2004) for example described her quest, as a woman with spina bifida, to have a child of her own. This journey in search for meaning, with several losses, physical pain and dehumanizing and humiliating experiences was also a celebration of sexual activity. A moment of resolution occurred when a number of parents shared a ceremony for those who had died on 9/11, an anniversary which coincided with the date of Neville-Jan's first miscarriage. In one article, Hoppes (2005a) described the death of his nephew, and his role in supporting family members decide what to do. He documented a range of activities including sharing meals, boating, attending baseball games, and helping the dying child's siblings maintain their lives. These activities were important in enabling people to cope with the event of the child's death.

In a second paper, Hoppes (2005b) described the family occupations associated with the death of his father. In the paper he recognized that being involved in the care for his father as his death got nearer prepared him for his own death, while caring for his mother facilitated his ability to deal with loss. Salmon (2006) described activities such as gardening with and making memory books about family events with her mother who was experiencing dementia. She found that the process of caring, though increasingly exhausting, was a necessary task that she had to accomplish in order to work through the process of separation from her mother as her dementia advanced. She also felt a need not only to engage in intense exercises as a means of seeking relief from the task of care giving, but eventually, to re-engage with aspects of herself which she had to neglect during the period of looking after her mother. All the above examples illustrate the importance of leisure and productive occupations performed with others, including caregiving, in providing meaning in peoples' lives

Conclusion

The findings from the literature review in this chapter suggest that in their journey in search for meaning, individuals are conveyed by culture, religion, folktales, and intellectual pursuits as vehicles. The sources of meaning include cultural and religious affiliations, relationships, and what people do (occupations) including work and leisure pursuits. The dimensions of meaning experienced from these sources include experience of oneself as having: self-worth; purpose in life; a sense of control of life circumstances through personal choices; and ability to act according to personal values. Relationships are ubiquitous as supreme sources of meaning in all the above discussed activities and dimensions of meaning. Therefore, in order for work, leisure, and intellectual pursuits to be ultimately meaningful, they have to occur in the context of meaningful family, intimate, and other social relationships. In the next chapter, the way in which people use occupations to tap into these sources and dimensions of meaning in various developmental stages as individuals progress through the life journey will be explored.

Apply the ideas discussed in Chapter 4

This exercise is designed to help your client be more cognizant of how he is eliciting meaning and experiencing its dimensions in his journey through life. Now, ask your client to take a few moments to reflect on his life journey and answer the following questions as exhaustively as he can.

1. **What are the sources of meaning in your client's life journey in his perspective?**

   1. Emotionally intense relationship(s);
   2. Work;
   3. Leisure activities;
   4. Affiliation to an idea system such as:
      a. Cultural traditions,
      b. Religion,
      c. Political ideology, etc.
   5. Something else

Guide your client to use a mind-map diagram to describe these sources of meaning in life as exhaustively as possible [e.g., if one source is an emotionally intense relationship, what is the nature of that relationship? Who is the other person involved in the relationship? What are her characteristics? What does your client do with this person, and how does she feel when with that person? Ask the client to repeat the above reflection for any other identified sources of meaning (i.e., work, leisure activities, etc.)]. The client can use artwork, poetry, or any other form of preferred self-expression to describe the sources of meaning in her life.

2. **Now ask the client to think about the manifestations of meaning in her life as a result of contact with the above identified sources of meaning.**

   These manifestations of meaning may be:
   1. A sense of self-worth;
   2. A sense of having a purpose in life;
   3. A sense of being in control of life circumstances, irrespective of what those circumstances might be;
   4. Ability to live out and/or express her values?

Many people may find it difficult to respond to such abstract directives. If your client is one of those people, you may guide her back to the mind map. Take an area, such as the person with whom your client has a relationship, or her leisure activities, and have her write out another mind map. When finished, for each associated word or idea, have the client develop a phrase. For each phrase, have her construct a sentence or a line of poetry, and then write this out on another sheet of paper. If preferred, the client can simply write these ideas down on sticky notes and tack them onto a paper on the wall. Ask the client not to be too careful or to worry about whether or not she is right. Aim for a maximum of ten phrases, constituting the first things that come into her mind. Ask her to cross things out, write in new phrases, and rearrange the text until she is satisfied. Then ask her to write it out again. Now, guide the client to decide which one is the best line, and take it out of the poem or piece. Ask the client to decide if the above process improves the piece for her. By doing this creative exercise, it may be easier to recognize and reflect on the dimensions of meaning, to appreciate what it is that gives the client a sense of self-worth or purpose, a sense of control, or a means of expressing values.

PART II OCCUPATIONS AND MEANING

In part I of this book we attempted to define the concept of meaning in life. Frankl's idea of the importance of meaning in life as a counter to meaninglessness experienced by people in our times was introduced. We discussed the idea of culture and other belief-defining institutions as vehicles that individuals use to pursue meaning in their journeys through life. We explored the sources and dimensions of meaning, and finally we examined how those sources and dimensions of meaning manifest in the various human developmental stages.

In part II of this book, which consists of chapter 5, we will examine more closely how occupations are used in each developmental stage to create meaning in life. Specific occupations that can be used by humans as a source of meaning in each stage of life will be suggested. This chapter will be a prerequisite to part III, in which more specific guidelines will be provided to help occupational therapists/scientists help their clients develop very specific plans to optimize meaning in life through occupational performance.

Chapter 5
The role of occupations in meaning-making in peoples' lives: A lifespan developmental perspective

Learning objectives

By the end of this chapter, the reader will be able to:

1. Explain how the sources and dimensions of meaning discussed in chapter 4 are related to the construct of participation
2. Articulate the relationships among participation, primary control, and agency
3. Identify occupations that individuals use to facilitate participation, a sense of primary control and agency, and subsequently experience their lives as meaningful at each developmental stage.
4. Help the client to identify occupations in which he/she participates that help him/her perform the specific role associated with the developmental tasks of his/her developmental stage, and how such participation enhances the sense of primary control, agency, and meaning in life.

Contents of this chapter

- Developmental and sociological lifespan perspectives of meaningful occupations
- Occupation, participation, primary role, primary control, agency, and life course developmental perspective
- Occupations as meaning-making/meaning-discovery instruments through agency, role fulfillment, and primary control at each developmental stage
- Relationships among occupations, the three sources of meaning, four dimensions of meaning, agency, primary role, and primary control at each developmental stage.

Introduction

In this chapter, the metaphor of the human search for meaning as a life-long journey will continue to be examined. The use of occupations as meaning-making instruments at each developmental stage in the journey will be explored. Before discussing how occupations are used developmentally for meaning-making, their relationship in general to the three sources and four dimensions of meaning identified in chapter four will be explored. The *three sources of meaning* were:

- establishment of *emotionally intense relationships*;
- engagement in meaningful *work and leisure activities*; and
- *adherence to idea systems.*

The *four dimensions of meaning* were:

- development of a sense of *self-worth*;
- having a sense of *purpose in life*;
- having a sense of *control* in life; and
- being able to express personal *values.*

In terms of occupational therapy and occupational science language, these sources and dimensions of meaning can be understood to constitute the human beings' need to engage in work and leisure activities (occupations) that help them to develop skills that make them: feel competent [develop a sense of self-worth and control in their lives]; feel connected to other people and to their communities [consistent with the notion of emotionally intense relationships as a source of meaning]; and establish a sense of meaning in their lives [have a sense of purpose in life] (Law, 2002). According to Law, the above delineated needs amount to engagement in occupations that enable one to participate in life, which she defined as "involvement or sharing, particularly in an activity" (p. 641). It seems then that participation through engagement in work and leisure occupations as defined by Law is a means by which people construct a meaningful existence by: establishing intense relationships; adhering to idea systems; having a sense of control in life and enhancing their self-worth; expressing personal values; and in essence establishing a sense of purpose in life.

The relationships among participation and the sources and dimensions of meaning as discussed in chapter four has been elaborated further by the World Health Organization [WHO] (2001) in the International Classification of Functioning, Disability and Health (ICF). According to the WHO, participation refers to involvement in life situations through engagement in occupations that make it possible for a person to: learn and apply knowledge; meet general task demands; communicate effectively with others; be mobile; complete self-care activities; engage in domestic life [what AOTA (2008a, 2008b) refers to as instrumental activities of daily living such as shopping, preparing meals, house-keeping, and taking care of others]; interact, form, and maintain relationships with others; be involved in major life areas such as pursuing informal education, going to school, obtaining and maintaining gainful employment, and participating in the community's economic life; and be involved in community, social, and civic life.

Law (2002) argued that participation could be achieved through performance of formal and informal occupations. Engagement in formal occupations is guided by well-articulated rules of performance geared towards achievement of specific goals. By contrast, informal occupations are initiated by individuals with little or no planning. In this chapter, we will examine occupations at every stage of development that humans use to make their lives meaningful by tapping into the sources and dimensions of meaning as defined above through participation. We will use the Lifespan developmental perspective as a way of identifying occupations that are the primary sources of meaning at every developmental stage in the human journey through life.

However, because human beings are complex, we realize that the lifespan developmental framework alone is not enough in helping us understand fully the types of occupations that make life meaningful for individuals at each developmental stage. Therefore, we will use the sociological lifespan perspective (Mayer, 2002, 2000) to provide insights into mutual transactions among the person, her biological, psychological, and sociological development and maturation, and the social context in which the person exists. This perspective will illuminate the interaction between the macro and micro factors that shape the human lifespan trajectory. In order to understand how occupations provide meaning to human beings at each developmental stage, we will also use the motivational theory of lifespan development (Hechhausen, 1999; Heckhausen, Schulz, & Wrosch, 2010; Heckhausen & Schulz, 1993). Below is a more detailed explanation of the above three theoretical frameworks and why they are suitable for helping us understand the process of meaning-making through occupational choices and performance at each developmental stage in the human life journey.

Lifespan developmental theories

The lifespan developmental theories explain how biological growth and psychological maturation influence valuation and choice of occupations and occupational roles that are seen by individuals as important. In this regard, we will use the work of developmental theorists such as Havighurst (1971), Erikson (1975, 1968, 1950), Levinson (1978), and Levinson and Levinson (1996) as a guide.

Life course theory

The life course theory (Mayer, 2002) will guide our understanding of the valuation, choice, performance, and meaning of occupations as a result of individual lives that are embedded:

> ...into social structures primarily in form of the partaking in social positions and roles, i.e., with their regard to their membership in institutional orders. The sociological study of the life course, therefore, aims at mapping, describing and explaining the synchronic and diachronic distribution of individual persons into social positions across the lifetime. (p. 2)

Using the life course (sociological) theory will help us clarify the social roles in which people participate throughout life that make their lives meaningful, and the occupations that make such participation possible. This clarification is important in explaining how occupations fit into the sources (engagement in *emotionally intense relationships* and *adhering to idea systems*) and dimensions (*self-worth*, *control*, expression of *values*) of meaning because the theoretical propositions of the framework address the above sources and dimensions.

The four primary propositions in this theoretical perspective are (Mayer, 2002):

1. One's life course is a transaction with the life courses of other people (i.e., this explains the importance of engaging in meaningful occupations that foster *relationships*) and social group as a whole (*connection to something larger than oneself*).
2. The life course consists of many dimensions including family, work, biological growth, and psychological maturation.
3. Life course is a product of one's actions (occupational performance) based on her individual experiences and available resources.
4. The way in which each person constructs his life course contributes to the reproduction and potential change of social structures. For example, one social structure that has changed in the recent past due to accumulation of individual actions is the increased concern by corporations about child care due to the need to accommodate more and more women who combine child rearing with formal employment.

Motivational theory of life-span development

Finally, the motivational theory of life-span development (Heckhausen et al., 2010) will help us understand how individuals value, choose, and perform occupations to achieve primary and secondary control in their lives. Primary control refers to the sense of agency that people experience due to the belief that they can achieve valued goals. Secondary control refers to goal adjustment that occurs when one realizes that she cannot achieve those goals. In other words, the motivational theory of lifespan development provides us with a way of understanding the "control" dimension of meaning based on the premise that "persons want to be masters of their own destinies: that they want to pursue their own goals and that they do so by exerting control over their environment" (Mayer, 2002, p. 13).

Role of occupations in participation at different stages of life

In infancy and early childhood

The three critical questions that will guide reflection in this section are: 1) What occupations are expected in infancy and childhood? 2) What level of mastery is expected in these occupations? 3) What skills are needed for that level of occupational mastery to be achieved? According to Havighurst (1971), the tasks of infancy and toddler stage (birth to three years) include learning how to hold things, crawl, walk, talk, and ingest solid foods. Thus, one may argue that in infancy, participation is primarily geared towards ensuring survival, which means acquiring nutrition, but also attaining increased mobility and therefore enhanced interaction with and exploration of the wider world. But according to Erikson (1950), in order to attain mastery of those tasks, the infant has to establish a sense of basic trust of the world as a safe and warm place, which subsequently gives him a sense of confidence necessary for further exploration of his environment and therefore a sense of increased autonomy. Therefore, the occupations of infancy consist of *relational and play activities* directed towards developing motor skills and a sense of trust and autonomy as described above. Such occupations involve, "mouthing, banging, dropping, and throwing objects" and developing increased, "independence in self-care tasks such as self-feeding and hand washing" (Davis & Polatajko, 2010, p. 142).

One of the key assurances an infant appears to need is that of a continued existence in the world. This explains the importance of staying within her mother's line of sight, or the mother returning a toy thrown out of view to the pram or cot (Winnicott, 1971). Winnicott's development of the object relations theory stemmed from the observation of the infant's capacity for representing relationships to the world through significant objects, such as the blanket or special toy which had to go everywhere she went. These objects enabled the child to make transitions because they represented a continuous and safe space inhabited by the child and her relationship with the mother from which she could explore new environments or situations. Often the need for this continuity was expressed by the child not allowing this transitional object for example to be washed because preservation of its smell and taste was very re-assuring to the infant.

The importance of continuity, as indicated by a desire for routine, is also apparent in other occupational dimensions in the infants' daily life. A child may demand that Mummy rather than Daddy always perform certain care functions, or that Mummy do certain things that the child knows he can do himself, but wants the security of her doing them. Routine can be important in enabling the child to explore the environment - for example visiting relatives or going on holiday may be a source of insecurity because the child is away from home, but might be less worrying if the same bedtime story is told to him. Gauvain (2001) suggested that a key part of the development of the child's capacities, including cognitive maturation probably resided in interactions with parents, and the parents' skills in perceiving and reacting appropriately to the needs of the child as much as in his innate capabilities.

Further, it has been observed that mothers tend to have more awareness of their children's needs and so generally seem to be able to provide greater security [or "scaffolding" according to Gauvain (2001, p. 169)] by finding a way of gaining the child's co-operation for task accomplishment. In summary, in infancy, the developmental tasks include: development of motor skills necessary to obtain nutrition and therefore to survive; attaining increased mobility and exploration of the immediate environment; and development of a sense of security, trust, and autonomy. Therefore, the primary occupational role of the infant as an active agent (Heckhausen et al., 2010) includes being able to initiate and manage motor tasks that cause events to happen, and relating to the caring adult in order to ensure safety. The infant's striving for primary control is achieved by engaging in occupational behaviour that results in rewards, such as throwing a toy over the cot so that the mother can commend her, pick it up, and bring it back, and smiling and vocalizing in order to receive a relational response from the caring adult.

In early childhood (ages 3 to 6 years), the child learns physical skills needed for games, has improved eye-hand coordination, and develops small muscle coordination so that now he can draw circles, pour liquid into a bowl, and button and unbutton clothes (Havighust, 1971). Control of elimination of body waste is also mastered. The child learns the differences between males and females, and is ready to learn to read. This is the age when many children begin school. Language skills develop rapidly. According to Erikson (1950), this is the stage in which the child develops initiative.

This is also the age at which the child begins experimenting with the roles that define the kind of person she imagines becoming as an adult. For example, Gauvain (2001) described how her daughter invited herself into her mother's activity of making a cake, a process which had to be slowed down to accommodate the child so as to ensure her successful participation. These early experiences are very important in determining the repertoire of occupational engagements a person may develop in later life. The time to make a cake, with its process slowed down to allow the child to participate was invested with meanings especially if the activity was presented to the child as 'fun', or as 'making a cake with Mum'. The product also had meaning for the child because she could talk proudly about 'a cake which I made with Mum'. This attention to the present relationship with others underpins the *human relationships* as a significant source of meaning at all ages because it allows reciprocation. As Berne (1964) suggested, some roles could be played out in games which invited participation, offering a chance for children to adopt appropriate or inappropriate roles. Such behaviour, learned through games in childhood, continues into adult life.

Also, in childhood, many opportunities for the development of occupational capacities occur in an organic way through everyday situations. Children naturally seek to investigate the world around them and to emulate the activities of their parents or siblings, and it follows that the richer the experiential world, the greater the potential for the child to recognise his potential and to discover and compensate for limitations. Freedom to *play* freely and to *use imagination* is critical at this stage of development. Resnick (2007) cautions us about the threat that educational methods in kindergarten with their emphasis on the acquisition of phonetics and other skills poses to creativity and free play. A sense of meaning through the experience of control and self-worth can only be achieved at this stage through engagement in occupations (*play activities*) involving free imagination using for example toys such as *wooden blocks, toy cars, and figures*. These occupations provide the children with a medium through which the real and imaginary worlds can be represented and through which solutions to physical problems can be found in collaboration with others in peer relationships.

Therefore, in early childhood, the developmental tasks include development of the gross and fine motor skills needed to perform *self-care activities* such as dressing, control and management of elimination activities, development of basic *reading skills*, and *beginning school*. Other tasks include understanding gender sex differences and imaginatively *enacting adult roles*. The role of the child in determining her developmental trajectory (agency) includes development of increased autonomy and sense of initiative. The occupations that the child uses to achieve a sense of primary control and therefore a sense of meaning and self-worth include: *self-care activities* such as dressing and undressing, brushing teeth, washing and drying face, setting the table, assisting with food preparation, etc.; *leisure activities* such as imaginative play and riding a bicycle; and *productive occupations* such as cutting with scissors, completing simple puzzles, using an eraser effectively, sharing toys, following rules, reading, and relating to peers (Davis & Polatajko, 2010).

This brings us to the later childhood. Gottfredson (1996, p. 189-191) suggested that early experiences influenced childrens' development of 'circumscription' principles through which they assessed their own capacities for particular occupations, including whether those occupations were realistically attainable. She described how children relinquished magical thinking about unrealistic career choices around the ages of 3 to 5 years, developed a more concrete awareness of adult gender roles between ages 6 and 8, and from the age of 9 acquired a sense of social value judgment, which by age 13 was more or less equivalent to an adult understanding of the status of certain careers.

According to Havighurst (1971), in later childhood (6-11 years), the developmental tasks were to develop even further physical skills needed for play, learn how to relate to peers, learn appropriate male and female social roles, achieve independence in all aspects of self-care, and begin developing an understanding of social group and institutional rules and norms. The child also transitioned from Kindergarten to grade school. Erikson (1950) stated that at this stage, the child developed a sense of industry, characterized by ability to work in cooperative activities with others, leading to a sense of competency. Based on the above discussion, it can be surmised that the primary control striving at this stage is to achieve *academic and sports competency*, and to be recognized and accepted by peers. To achieve this control and subsequent sense of self-worth, and therefore to experience a sense of meaning, the child engages in the following occupations: *leisure occupations* such as playing card games that require cognitive skills and decision-making, making and giving gifts to valued people in her life, watching television and listening to music; *activities of daily living* such as demonstrating appropriate table manners during meals; and *productive activities* such as completing school work and competently engaging in sports activities as required.

In adolescence

According to Havighurst (1971), in adolescence (ages 12 to 18 years), individuals begin to relate to peers of the same age in both sexes in more mature ways. They begin to identify more with masculine or feminine roles, to accept and to use their physical bodies effectively, and to develop emotional independence from parents and other adults. Biologically and emotionally, they are preparing for adult relationships and family life. They begin to develop a value system as a basis for ethical frameworks to guide their behaviour, and begin striving towards responsible social behaviour. This is the stage in which according to Eriksson (1975), the individual seeks to establish a sense of identity.

One of the major tasks of adolescence is to begin contemplating a *career and assumption of adult roles*. Whereas in earlier stages most children learn social rules about the *appropriateness* of certain occupational choices, in adolescence they begin to focus more on how their abilities and personalities can be aligned with the career opportunities available to them commensurate with their family needs. They begin to develop an understanding of the compromises they must make in order to increase the likelihood of realising their aspirations. Gottfredson (1996) suggests that compromises that occur at this stage involve: narrowing of expectations for anticipated career choices to focus more on options that are realistically achievable or that are congruent with social status; realizing that desired achievements may not be attainable through careers - but may be attainable through pursuit of other occupations outside work, much as we explored in chapter two in relation to the second author's experiences prior to becoming an occupational therapist, and the exploration of worker-writer narratives.

Gottfredson asserts that on the whole people are not very willing to compromise on gender-related occupational role choices. For example, men will choose careers of lower social prestige rather than higher status 'female' jobs. Women are more flexible but will avoid clearly defined 'male' type work roles. The significance of this gender role delineation is apparent in the profession of occupational therapy where a narrow identification of the profession with females may have significantly limited the effectiveness of efforts to encourage male entrants into the profession (currently, in Europe, Australia, and North America, males constitute only about 5% of occupational therapists).

Gottfredson's theory is that experiential issues affect these circumscriptions from early developmental stages because children develop increasingly complex assessments of their self-worth, social status, and the possibilities open to them quite early in life. Some of these judgments may be taken for granted. Also, the assessments may alter as changes in social situations produce unanticipated opportunities, or require the intervention of others to make options that a person may have been unable to perceive or for which she may have ruled herself out available. Changes in peer perceptions of gender prescriptions may also impact the way individuals evaluate career options available to them since as Passmore (2003) found in one study, the development of self-worth in adolescence depends on the regular experience of competencies which are affirmed through peer relationships.

Leisure occupations are also an important part of the adolescent developmental stage. In Western countries, leisure occupations take up a significant part of adolescence time, and so it is an important occupational category in which young people need to be able to access positive opportunities for discovering and developing competence in social, educational, behavioural, and physical skills. Therefore, the developmental tasks of adolescents include: establishment of identity and a value system; preparation for and choice of a career; assumption of adult roles; development of emotional maturity; and learning to engage in more mature relationships. The role of the adolescent in contributing to lifespan developmental trajectory includes developing competency in relating to others socially, and acquiring skills necessary for transitioning into future career and adult roles. The adolescent's primary control striving is to be accepted by peers, to be successful in romantic relationships, and to be treated as an adult.

According to Davis and Polatajko (2010), the occupations that the adolescent uses to achieve the above objectives include: leisure occupations such as hobbies, out of school sports activities, and watching television or listening to music; productive occupations such as obtaining and holding a job, earning and spending money; instrumental activities of daily living such as routine household repairs and maintenance; and social occupations including repaying money borrowed from others.

In emerging adulthood

Emerging adulthood is the stage immediately following adolescence but prior to the assumption of adult responsibilities. It extends between the ages of 18 and 25 years and may go on to 29 years of age. This stage is characterized by a focus on the self, self-exploration, and examination of possibilities (Tanner & Arnett, 2009). It results from a need for extended education and subsequent delay in transition to a career and family responsibilities. As a species, human beings have developed a longer period of physical dependency on mature members of the species than any other animal (Gauvain, 2001). The age of dependency has extended to young adults within the relatively recent social history - for example as the age for marriage has been extended, the expectation for young people to leave school and to engage in the workforce has been postponed to the late 20s or even early 30s. Facing over more than a decade and a half of continued dependency, children and parents have had to re-negotiate relationships in a changing occupational situation in which both child and adult are progressing in capabilities, and in a family environment which may involve older or younger siblings at different developmental stages.

Notice though that as Tanner and Arnett (2009) acknowledge, emerging adulthood is primarily a middle class phenomenon because it is the middle class and rich family children that tend to attend college for an extended period of time. As mentioned in chapter 5, studies need to be conducted to determine cross-cultural and within-culture relevance of this developmental stage. None the less, other reasons why this stage of development has resulted include the changed roles of women, so that now they can develop a career and do not have to be married at age 18 and begin bringing up children; and increased tolerance for premarital sex such that people do not need to get married to enjoy sexual activities (sexual activities among young adults now on average begin about 10 years before marriage).

Further, the primary developmental tasks at this stage are re-centering and identity formation/stabilization (Schwartz, Cote, & Arnette, 2005; Tanner & Arnett, 2009). Recentering is characterized by the following four developments:

1. Individual relationships and roles shift from a state of dependence to a state of shared power and reciprocity. This happens through renegotiation of one's relationship with parents as explained earlier, allowing increased assumption of financial responsibility and decision-making while at the same time receiving support from the parents.
2. Engagement in temporary and transitory relationships and roles. The individual explores a variety of relationships and roles as he searches for opportunities to satisfy work and love life.
3. Final commitment to adult roles and responsibilities. This includes finally settling down on a career, marriage or some other type of partnership, and becoming a parent.

In essence, emerging adulthood is a time of setting and prioritizing life goals.

Stable identity formation on the other hand is based on being proactive by actively planning goals that contribute to determination of a desired life course trajectory (being agentic). There are two paths to identity formation (Schwartz et al., 2005):

1. Default individualization – In this path, the individual makes decisions on impulse and is easily influenced by what seems to be fashionable trends, rather than engaging in activities that are likely to lead to personal growth. The individual may therefore end up ill prepared for life roles and responsibilities.
2. Developmental individualization – the person engages in continued, deliberate growth, by choosing to take advantage of opportunities for skill acquisition and personal growth, rather than following the path of least resistance (typically what seems fashionable in the moment).

Developmental individualization requires agency on the part of the individual. By agency is meant "the belief that one is in control of one's decisions and is responsible for their outcomes, and the confidence that one will be able to overcome obstacles that impend one's progress along one's chosen life course" (Schwartz et al., p. 207). In their study, Schwartz et al. found that, "those emerging adults who utilize default individualization strategies score relatively low in ego strength [suggesting lack of adequate will], self-esteem, and life purpose [the sense that their lives are purposeful and meaningful] and they appear to have a lack of commitment to a set of goals, values, and beliefs that would provide a basis for guiding their way through the exceptionally unstructured years of emerging adulthood" (p. 224). Thus the meaning-making model discussed in chapter 6 might be particularly appropriate for use with individuals at this developmental stage. It is a way of helping them to develop a mission that becomes the basis for goal-formulation providing the needed action-oriented focus and therefore agency in their lives.

Given the above discussion, the major developmental tasks of the emerging adulthood include re-centering and stable identity formation. Other tasks include forming friendships, academic pursuits (as part of skill acquisition and personal growth consistent with developmental individualization), seeking romance, and work exploration. The person's primary agentic role [consistent with the motivational theory (Heckhausen et al., 2010)] is to make choices consistent with skill development and personal growth so that she is prepared to transition to work and other adult responsibilities. The occupations that enable the individual to fulfill this role and therefore to experience meaning in life include *dating* and other activities that would eventually result in sexual satisfaction, *formal education participation*, *informal personal education participation* (seeking knowledge in personally identified areas of interest), *employment seeking and acquisition*, *engaging in community, family, and peer activities* (American Occupational Therapy Association [AOTA], 2014).

In adulthood

Adulthood begins somewhere in the late 20s and covers the entire period of the 30s. The main task in this developmental stage is to establish oneself by committing and establishing roots in society, and becoming one's own person (Levinson, 1978). According to Havighurst (1971), the developmental tasks of this stage include selecting a mate (some people get married), learning to live with a partner (such as a wife), starting a family and rearing children, home management, establishing oneself in a career, fulfilling civic responsibilities such as paying taxes and participating in the political discourse, and finding and participating in a social group.

It is important to note however that due to recent changes in social structure due to globalization, increased mobility, and work environment, the validity of the above outlined developmental tasks may be in question. It has been observed for instance that the way careers evolve has dramatically changed in recent years (Sullivan, 1999). The traditional linear model of career progression in which success is measured by promotions and pay raise within organizations may not work anymore. Workers in current times may need to work two or more part time jobs, with increased job responsibilities, and fewer chances for promotion. Therefore, self-establishment in a stable career is one of those developmental tasks of adulthood that may need to be re-conceptualized.

Irrespective of the changes however, it can be argued that the adult person's role as an agent in determining his/her own life-span course (primary control) would be to: *commit to a mate* with whom to spend life; establish and bring up a *family* (for those so inclined); establish himself in a *career* in some way; and become a *participating, contributing member of society*. The occupations that enable one to fulfill the above role and therefore to experience meaning in life include *child rearing*, *finding a job* (career), engaging in *community activities* and fulfilling civil obligations, engaging in *family, and social activities.*

In midlife

Midlife is often characterized as a transition stage between adulthood and older age (Erikson, 1975; Jung, 1971; Levinson, 1978). However, the chronological age when this transition occurs is not clear. Depending on various authors' points of view, it could range anywhere from the 30s to the 70s (Lachman & James, 1997). For a 20 year old, it is between 30 and 60. For people in their 50s, it is between 45 and 70. The average seems to be between 35 and 65. What is more important though is that middle age is generally conceptualized to consist of certain characteristics. People's level of energy and physical strength begin to be compromised, so that they are likely to be concerned about their health in general. Muscle strength, especially in the back and lower extremities is compromised so that they increasingly experience difficulties maintaining balance and rising from sit to stand (Kuh et al., 2006).

Developmentally, according to Eriksson (1975), at this stage people are negotiating the tasks of generativity (the sense that they are productive and contributing effectively to society) versus stagnation (a sense that they have stopped growing and progressing). Healthy development denotes cultivating the feeling that one is productive and nurturing. While people at this stage have accumulated some expertise and experienced success at work, and have satisfying social and family lives, they now have a desire to nurture others, and to contribute to the development of younger generations. That is why one of the tasks of individuals at this stage, according to Levinson (1978), is to mentor younger people both at work and in other spheres of life. They are also concerned about the well-being and success of their children, as well as the well-being of their aging parents. At the same time, they are thinking about their own future and are preparing for retirement among other things.

Therefore, the developmental tasks of this age include: maintaining a comfortable home; trying to assure a secure financial and emotional future; sharing household responsibilities; cultivating emotional closeness to the spouse/life partner; staying close to grown children and their families (or parenting adolescent children, or launching young adult children); keeping in touch with/taking care of aging parents; keeping in touch with siblings and their families, with other relatives, and with friends; participating in the community life, and focusing on internal growth through development of spirituality or philosophical/social pursuits. The primary control (agentic) roles [primary sources of meaning] (Heckhausen et al., 2010) for individuals in this developmental stage include enhancement of their sense of generativity, re-evaluation of values, development of new interests, and preparation for transition to retirement. The occupations that they use to accomplish the above roles successfully include: *mentoring* younger workers; *child-rearing* (parenting adolescent children or launching young adult children); *home management*; *job performance*; preparing for and adjusting to *retirement*; *leisure exploration*; *family role* performance; and *community participation* (AOTA, 2014).

In older adulthood

After midlife, individuals transition to the older adult stage (roughly 60 years of age and over). At this point, one has already retired or is in the process of retiring from paid employment. However, note that with the changing labour market (Sullivan, 1999), this may no longer be the case. There are many people who continue engaging in paid employment until they are 70 years of age or even older. None the less, according to Erikson (1986), the older adult stage involves the individual either developing ego integrity, where he looks back at his entire life and experiences a sense of satisfaction, or despair where the person looks back at his life and sees a wasted existence. If the earlier stages have been negotiated satisfactorily, the person feels that he has lived a good life, has contributed something significant to society, and has met most of his life goals.

Given the above described struggle between a sense of integrity and despair, the individual is in a state of self-evaluation. One tends to look back at her life and tries to evaluate how she has lived. Older adults also tend to adjust their goals with a realistic awareness that time is running out and some of the goals will not be met. This is necessary considering that one of the themes in this stage is loss: retirement from the workforce (loss of paid employment), death (loss) of a spouse, declining health, loss of physical strength, etc. (University of California San Francisco Nursing Department, 2001). This experience of loss calls for adaptation to the current reality, and such adaptation includes a re-appraisal of goals and dreams. However, older adults also continue to seek the experience of being in control and continuing to engage in society (Russell, n.d.). That is why the need for older adults to maintain agency through participation as a way of maintaining health and security is inherent in the notion of 'active aging' as defined by the World Health Organization (WHO, 2002).

Given the above discussion, the developmental tasks of older adults include being financially responsible, adapting to changes in their lives, and continued engagement in society through participation, or what Eriksson (1986) calls *vital involvement.* Therefore, engagement in occupations that help complete the above tasks is a significant means of exercising primary control and therefore a source of meaning for older adults. Such occupations include those that facilitate: quality *relationships* with other people, particularly younger generations and peers [what in occupational science have been called co-occupations (Pickens & Pizur-Barnekow, 2009; Price & Stephenson, 2009) such as participating in family board games]; *reminiscence* (for example writing an autobiography, writing family history, scrap-booking, i.e., narrating family history through photos and artifacts); *staying connected* to society (engagement in occupations that are valued by society, such as *volunteering*); continued *independence and autonomy* (for example by learning how to use a computer to do on-line banking thus avoiding the need for transportation to the bank); adaptation to technological changes; and maintenance of cognitive functioning (Russel, n.d.).

Conclusion

In this chapter, we explored the theme of the human life as a journey, in which the person seeks nourishment from various sources of meaning in order to make it through the journey in a healthy, fulfilling manner. We discussed the idea that there are significant sources and dimensions of meaning at each stage, and introduced the argument that such sources and dimensions of meaning are closely connected to the theme of participation as defined by the World Health Organization, and primary control as proposed by lifespan developmental theorists. We argued that occupations that would help an individual construct meaning at each stage of her life are those that enhance participation and primary control (the sense that one can influence the direction of her development through actions that make it possible to meet personal goals, also known as agency). Therefore, for each developmental stage, we identified typical occupations in which individuals do/could participate in order to exercise primary control and therefore experience life as meaningful. The summary of the primary roles associated with each developmental stage and occupations that enhance individual ability to fulfill those roles is presented in Table 5-1 below.

Table 5-1. Occupations that are used by individuals at each developmental stage to facilitate participation, achievement of primary control, and construction of meaning in life

Developmental tasks	Primary control strategies (role of individual as an agent)	Occupations used to achieve primary control and enhance meaning
Developmental stage: Infancy		
· Development of motor skills · Increased mobility and environmental exploration · Development of sense of security, trust, and autonomy	· Initiating and managing motor tasks necessary to cause events to happen · Initiating behaviour needed to relate to caring adults	· Throwing toys in the presence of a caring adult · Smiling and vocalizing
Developmental stage: Early childhood		
· Learning physical skills needed to play games · Improved eye-hand co-ordination · Increased muscle coordination · Control of body waste · Learning gender differences · Beginning kindergarten · Improved language skills	· Learning adult behaviour through imaginative play	· Play activities involving toys · Self-care activities (dressing, brushing teeth, setting table, etc.) · Cutting with scissors · Completing puzzles · Using eraser effectively · Sharing toys · Reading · Relating to peers

Table 5-1. Continued

Developmental tasks	Primary control strategies (role of individual as an agent)	Occupations used to achieve primary control and enhance meaning
Developmental stage: Late childhood		
· Continued development of motor skills · Learning how to relate to peers · Learning gender roles · Achieving independence in self care · Understanding rules and norms	· Achieving academic and sports competency · Being recognized by peers	· Leisure occupations (e.g. card games) · Making and giving gifts to valued people · Watching television · Listening to music · Activities of daily living such as observing dining etiquette · Competently completing academic and sports activities
Developmental stage: Adolescence		
· Establishing a sense of identity · Contemplating adult roles · Preparing for future career · Developing emotional maturity · Learning to engage in more mature relationships	· Developing competency in relating to others socially · Learning skills necessary to transition to adult roles	· Leisure occupations such as hobbies, sports, watching television, and listening to music · Productive occupations such as obtaining a job, earning and spending money · House maintenance · Engaging in social occupations

Table 5-1. Continued

Developmental tasks	Primary control strategies (role of individual as an agent)	Occupations used to achieve primary control and enhance meaning
Developmental stage: Emerging adulthood		
· Re-centering · Identity formation/stabilization · Forming friendships · Academic pursuits · Romantic engagements · Work exploration	· Actively setting and prioritizing life goals · Developing skills to ensure personal growth	· Dating and other courtship activities · Formal education participation · Informal personal education participation · Seeking and acquiring employment · Engaging in community, family, and peer activities
Developmental stage: Adulthood		
· Selecting a life mate · Learning to live with a partner · Starting a family and bringing up children · Home management · Establishing oneself in career · Fulfilling civic responsibilities · Finding and participating in a social group	· Committing to another person, establishing a family, establishing oneself in a career, and becoming a participating member of the community	· Child rearing · Finding a job and establishing a career · Engaging in community activities · Engaging in family activities · Engaging in social activities

Table 5-1. Continued

Developmental tasks	Primary control strategies (role of individual as an agent)	Occupations used to achieve primary control and enhance meaning
Developmental stage: Midlife		
· Maintaining a comfortable home · Seeking emotional and financial security · Sharing household responsibilities · Relating to spouse, children, and parents · Relating to siblings, other relatives, and friends · Seeking internal growth	· Enhancing a sense of generativity, re-assessment of values, development of new interests, and preparation for retirement	· Mentoring younger generations · Child rearing · Home management · Job performance · Preparing for retirement · Leisure exploration · Family role performance · Community participation

Table 5-1. Continued

Developmental tasks	Primary control strategies (role of individual as an agent)	Occupations used to achieve primary control and enhance meaning
Developmental stage: Older adult		
· Maintaining financial responsibility · Adapting to change · Continuing to engage in society	· Continued participation in life through meaningful occupations	· Engaging in co-occupations (to enhance relationships) · Reminiscing through occupations such as writing autobiographies and family histories · Engaging in occupations that are valued by society · Learning skills necessary to maintain independence and autonomy · Engaging in cognitively challenging activities

Application of ideas discussed in Chapter 5

The purpose of the following two exercises is to help your client personalize the information in this chapter by reflecting on the developmental stages of some people in his life, and the stage-specific occupations that they use to create meaning in their lives. The client will also reflect on his own current developmental stage, developmental tasks in that stage and how he manages the direction of his future development through participation in meaningful occupations, and therefore how he can create meaning in life through this form of agency. Now guide your client in completing the exercise on Figure 5-1 overleaf.

Appraisal of each person's success in accomplishing developmental tasks through occupations to optimize meaning in life

For each person listed in figure 5-1, ask the client to write down a statement or two about the extent to which the person is managing the stage-specific developmental tasks. What occupations does the client think that this person could perform routinely in order to accomplish developmental tasks more effectively and therefore to experience optimal meaning in her life?

Developmental stages and agency occupations for the clients

Now, ask the client to think about her life and to answer the following questions:

1. In what developmental stage is the client?
2. What are her current developmental tasks?
3. What does she perceive as the primary role in determining the future direction of her developmental trajectory?
4. What are the occupations in which she currently participates or could participate in order to determine more effectively the desired developmental trajectory?
5. To what extent is engagement in those occupations related to how meaningful the client experiences life to be right now? Ask her to explain

Figure 5-1. Matrix of the developmental tasks of people close to the client's family, and the occupations they use to exert control over their life trajectories

Developmental stages and agency occupations for significant people in the client's life
Ask the client to choose five close people in his/her life (family members and/or friends). For each person, have the client enter the following information in the matrix below:

Name of the person	Developmental Stage	Developmental Tasks	Primary Control Strategies (The person's role as an Agent in shaping his/her developmental trajectory)	Occupations used to Achieve Primary Control and Enhance Meaning in life

PART III ACTION

In this part of the book, we present guidelines for the culminating experience of occupational therapy/occupational science intervention. The whole purpose of therapy is to create change that makes clients' lives more fulfilling and meaningful. This part of the book provides tools towards that end. In the previous chapters, the construct of meaning has been discussed as it may be conceptualized from multiple perspectives. We have examined typical ways in which people use occupations to construct meaningful existence using the perspectives of English worker-writers to provide the context for that understanding. The role of occupations in constructing meaningful existence at every stage of life in the human life-span development has been examined. In chapter 6, we briefly discuss the Instrumentalism in Occupational Therapy (IOT) model and propose a step by step process that therapists can use to guide clients in enhancing meaning in their lives through daily occupations. It may be useful for students and therapists to try and apply the proposed procedures to enhance meaning in their own lives through their daily occupational choices and performance. That experiential learning could help them develop insights that would make them more effective in using the same process with their clients.

Chapter 6
Guidelines for meaning-making through daily occupations

Learning objectives

By the end of this chapter, the reader will be able to:

1. Explain the theoretical propositions and clinical guidelines of the Instrumentalism in Occupational Therapy (IOT) theoretical conceptual practice model
2. Demonstrate ability to use the model's assessment and intervention guidelines to help clients identify and engage in occupations that optimize a sense of meaning in life
3. Explain available empirical evidence supporting the clinical effectiveness of strategies identified in the IOT practice guidelines in helping clients achieve desired goals

Contents of this chapter

- Guidelines for creating/discovering meaning in life through experience afforded by occupational choices
- Instrumentalism in Occupational Therapy (IOT) as a source of theoretical guidelines for meaning-making through occupations
- Life aspirations as articulated in a personal mission statement as a compass for meaning-making
- Personal mission as a way of exercising agency, primary control, and acting in accordance with the three sources and four dimensions of meaning
- Identifying and defining life aspirations through a personal mission statement as a first step in meaning-making
- Choosing occupations to help clients achieve life aspirations
- Evaluating performance of occupations associated with aspirations in life
- Setting goals to facilitate needed occupational performance changes
- Continued re-assessment and adjustment of plan for change

Introduction

In her exhortation to occupational therapists to re-integrate themselves in mental health practice, Stoffel (2013), the then President-Elect of the American Occupational Therapy Association (AOTA) wrote that:

> Occupational therapy practitioners have much to offer recovery-oriented systems of care *given their expertise in helping people live meaningful lives* and pursue healthy daily routines. (p. 144, emphasis ours)

Stoffel's sentiments are consistent with the theme of this book, which is that occupational therapists/scientists can use their knowledge of the nature and health enhancing characteristics of occupations to help people in general construct meaningful lives through conscious choice and engagement in daily occupations. However, in chapter one, the definition of 'meaning' was found to be elusive because people attribute it to events in unique ways. What is meaningful could be that which: is consistent with survival (existential perspective); provides a means of connecting to a higher being such as God, and thus increasing a sense of perfection and eternity in an individual's mundane and finite life; and/or contributes to achievement of personally valuable goals. Meaningful life was defined as, 'a life of active engagement in projects of worth, which might involve such things as moral or intellectual accomplishments, relationship with family and friends, or artistic/creative enterprises' (Paul, Miller, & Paul, 1997, p. xii). It was also defined as a life that is experienced as providing coherence, a chance to be creative, and a sense of being in control.

In chapter two, this definition was further elaborated using the findings from a study by Ikiugu et al. (2012) in which the autobiographical writings of members of the Federation of Worker-Writers and Community Publishing (FWWCP) were analyzed. Ikiugu et al. found that these worker-writers made meaning in their lives by engaging in occupations that they saw as contributing to a definition of their identities, connecting to other people, connecting to causes larger than themselves, having a sense of coherence, and using their creativity. These findings fitted very well with the definition of meaning in chapter one in which meaning was conceptualized as resulting from a life of intellectual accomplishments, relationships with family members (connecting to other people), and engaging in creative/artistic activities. In chapters 3 to 5, the search for meaning was metaphorically compared to a journey (or quest), from birth through death. It was suggested that the vehicles used in this journey were the culture (including religious affiliations), and philosophical and scientific inquiry. Lifespan developmental stages could be analogically compared to stations, bus stages, ports, or airports along the path in the journey. At each station there are specific tasks to be accomplished. These tasks are accomplished through engagement in related occupations, and this process of accomplishing the tasks becomes the source of meaning.

The above discussion suggests that experience and choice are clearly components of the process of making meaning, and the outcomes are specific to each individual. These variables (experience and choice) have to be accounted for in any guidelines for creating meaning in life through occupations. In this chapter, we will first introduce a theoretical conceptual practice model which underpins the suggested guidelines. The specific practice guidelines will be described step by step, including: how to help individuals identify and define their life aspirations; choose occupations to help them achieve those aspirations; evaluate themselves on performance of those occupations; set goals to facilitate needed occupational performance changes; and re-evaluate themselves on a regular basis to determine how well they are progressing towards their aspirations.

Instrumentalism in Occupational Therapy (IOT)

Instrumentalism in Occupational Therapy (IOT)is a theoretical guide to meaning-making through daily occupations

Frankl (1992) argued that the human being is a holistic mind/body/spirit unity, with a basic need that he referred to as the 'will to meaning' (Elekes, 2011, p. 84). He further proposed that creating meaning is a personal responsibility and can be achieved by using one's creativity to serve other human beings. Meaning is achieved through connection with the world and with other people, substantial contribution to the world, experience of love and joy in life, maintenance of a positive attitude in the face of unavoidable suffering, and striving towards self-transcendence (Frankl, 1992), a kind of forgetting oneself in order to serve a greater cause and/or another person (Elekes, 2011). This view is consistent with the discussion in chapter 5 in which it became increasingly apparent that occupations that help people create meaning in their lives are primarily those that enhance participation and primary control at each stage of human development. Primary control refers to the sense that individuals can influence the course of their development by using their creativity to work towards personal goals. The Instrumentalism in Occupational Therapy (IOT) theoretical conceptual practice model (Ikiugu 2007, 2004a, 2004b, 2004c, or a later version of it (Modified Instrumentalism in Occupational Therapy, MIOT: see Ikiugu, 2011, 2008; Tupe, 2013), can be used to provide guidelines to help people to identify and engage in such occupations.

The IOT/MIOT framework was developed as a theoretical conceptual practice model consistent with occupational therapy's basic professional values and philosophical underpinnings. Ikiugu (2001, see also Ikiugu & Schultz, 2006) concluded that the philosophy of American pragmatism, particularly Dewey's (Kennedy, 1996) notion of instrumentalism, applied to occupational therapy practice because it denoted that the mind and its activities (thinking, problem-solving, inquiry, artistic endeavors, etc.) are tools, like any others, that human beings use to shape the environment so that it is conducive to their survival as a species. Dewey's argument is consistent with occupational therapy's historical focus on the mind as a primary point of intervention (Ikiugu, 2010, 2007). He makes the point that just as people have to learn how to use other tools (we learn how to operate a computer so that we can use it to write, communicate and perform other functions), they also need to learn how to use their minds effectively. This learning enables people to use their minds properly for the benefit of their well-being and the good of all humanity.

Ikiugu (2004a, 2004b, 2004c) decided to use the construct of instrumentalism as the cornerstone for a new theoretical conceptual practice model that was grounded on the principles of the philosophy of pragmatism. However, a philosophical orientation only provides a profession with identity and basic assumptions, including the logical basis of those assumptions (Ikiugu & Schultz, 2006). Philosophical principles by themselves cannot be operationalized for application to address the profession's domains of concern (Mosey, 1996). Therefore, a scientific theory was needed to provide basic constructs to the newly proposed theoretical conceptual practice model. Since Charles Darwin's theory of evolution was central to the development of pragmatism (Dewey, 1910), Ikiugu considered using it to provide a theoretical framework for the model. However, a further review of the literature revealed a new scientific discipline, complexity/chaos/dynamical systems theory, which seemed to be an improved version of Darwin's evolutionism (Ikiugu, 2007, 2004a, 2004b, 2004c), and therefore more suited as an explanatory framework for an occupational human being. Accordingly, to develop the IOT model, Ikiugu borrowed constructs from the philosophy of pragmatism, dynamical systems theory, and a variety of relevant psychological theories, primarily cognitive-behavioral psychology [because of its unique suitability in helping clients clarify beliefs guiding their actions, and therefore its consistence with the notion of 'beliefs as a rule for action' (Ikiugu, 2011, p. 114) as proposed by the originator of pragmatism, Charles Sanders Peirce (1955)].

Theoretical core of the IOT Model

The basic premise of IOT is that the occupational human being is a complex dynamical adaptive system. This means that a human being is in dynamic interaction with the environment through engagement in occupations. This dynamic interaction, which results largely from beliefs about self, others, and the environment (Ikiugu, 2007, 2004b) leads to the emergence of both physical and social change and subsequent adaptation. A person can consciously decide to act in such a way that he is optimally adaptive. Individuals may adapt their occupational routines to be consistent with a vision of the legacy that they want to create in life. In the perspective of the IOT, a personal mission statement specifies the components of a principled life involving personally satisfying family relationships, social relationships, work, and community participation (Ikiugu, 2007). Thus, living a principled life based on a clearly articulated personal mission in life would involve connectedness with one's family and social peers, satisfying work, and connection to an entity that is larger than oneself (such as one's cultural institutions, community, or a particular cause). Such living would be consistent with Frankl's (1992) definition of a meaningful life as we have discussed it in earlier chapters. It would also be consistent with Erikson's (1975) notion that the most important task in midlife is to create a sense of generativity. Creating a desired legacy in life ensures this sense of generativity. Later in life (older adult stage), the legacy leads to the ability to look back on life and feel a sense of fulfillment (sense of ego-integrity), and subsequent feelings of wisdom rather than regret, bitterness, and despair. Ikiugu (2007) defined adaptation as constituting living a life that is consistent with such a personal mission, and therefore in that sense, living a meaningful life. Based on this definition, maladaptation may be characterized as consisting of a daily occupational routine that is not consistent with a vision of one's mission in life, therefore leading to a possible feeling of lack of the sense that one's life has coherence, purpose, and meaning.

Generally, over time, people develop repertoires of occupations which relate to their environmental context. These repertoires consist of a dynamic which is repeated, perhaps with variations, over a person's occupational life trajectory. The effect is that a person remains true to his or herself, and the resulting life constitutes a trajectory through time that is constant or self-similar, in which occupation mediates the dynamic interaction of the individual with her environment (Ikiugu, 2005; Ikiugu & Rosso, 2005). Thus the occupational repertoire constitutes a life-path of daily occupational routines that when analyzed on a small scale reveals patterns which are similar to those of the entire trajectory covering a large time span of a person's life. Therefore, by examining a small part of a person's narrative, one can make an assessment regarding the state of adaptiveness or maladaptiveness of the entire life path. The trajectory is also sensitive to initial (or local) conditions. This means that making small changes in one's actions 'guided by the mind and will' to borrow from the famous statement by Reilly (1962) can result in big differences in the direction of the person's life path.

In other words, when individuals make small adjustments in their thoughts about themselves, other people, and the world, these small changes in cognitive perspective result in corresponding adjustment in their mundane occupational choices and performance, and this may lead to big differences in their feelings about meaning in life. This point is best illustrated by Hasselkus (2002) in her example of how a decision to incorporate her dental hygienist's advice to floss her teeth every day resulted in alteration of her wider occupational routine and a subsequent change in her experiences in life. In her reflection on the effect of this small change in her life, Hasselkus concluded:

> And so it is with all the occupational events of our lives – the small stuff and the big stuff of life contribute to the *development of each of us across the life span*. New ventures shift the balance of our days, and new ventures shift the nature of our inner selves. Possibilities that are taken on inevitably result in *accommodations in other aspects of our lives as we continually seek to balance the actual with the possible.* (p. 68, emphasis added)

Although in this statement she does not refer to the dynamical systems theory, Hasselkus' experience is a good illustration of the notion of sensitivity to local conditions in complexity theory. She explains the big differences in her occupational life trajectory that resulted from small changes in routine as the system accommodated the changes that she made by balancing 'the actual with the possible'. To guide the step-by-step process of creating meaningful existence through occupational performance, Constructs derived from the IOT model will be supplemented by ideas borrowed from the work of Mindell (2002, 2001, 1995, 1982). Mindell was a Jungian analyst who developed his own approach to therapy, known as Process-Oriented Psychology, in which he combined ideas from Jungian analysis, physics, Taoism, and Eastern healing traditions. He specializes in dream-work, working with people in relationships, group dynamics, and conflict resolution. Ideas borrowed from his work will be used to guide self-exploration that is necessary in examining personal beliefs that guide actions, before a mission statement geared towards legacy creation can be established.

Guidelines for meaning-making through daily occupational performance

Based on the theoretical core as explained above, the IOT/MIOT guidelines seek to operationalize the following process:

1. *belief establishment* (based on the premise that since the mind is a tool for shaping the environment, and beliefs are the fuel that energizes the mind, then one must cultivate beliefs that are consistent with the kind of physical and social environment that he/she perceives to be the best for supporting a personally meaningful life);
2. *action* (identification of occupations that would help individuals actualize their beliefs about self, others, and the environment, setting of goals to ensure effective performance of those occupations, and commitment to performance of the occupations to achieve those goals); and
3. *consequence appraisal* (evaluating consequences of one's occupational performance on an on-going basis and making adjustments accordingly; in other words learning from life experiences in order to optimize meaning in life).

Belief establishment

The first step in developing a strategy for meaning-making through daily occupational performance is to examine the beliefs that guide occupational choices and performance. This could begin with 'inner-work' (Mindell, 1995) to help the individual increase self-understanding. This self-exploration is based on the idea that without self-awareness, transformational visions cannot be truly formulated. People often engage in actions because they sense the need to change circumstances in their lives. However, peoples' actions do not always create the changes that they seek, and sometimes make things worse. For example, some individuals may want to lose weight because they realize that maintaining a healthy body/mass index is crucial to good health and the ability to work towards other life goals. Consequently they may put themselves on a strict diet, but after a few weeks, they may find that they have actually gained weight. They may then get frustrated and give up.

According to Mindell (1995), the changes people try to create in the world often fail to work because of a lack in sufficient awareness of their motives and how the changes fit in with their entire life circumstances. This lack of awareness not only prevents change, but can make our problems even worse. Mindell observed that the only way to create true, enduring change is to begin by increasing awareness of the underlying dynamics of the processes that guide our belief formation (including forms of psychic self-oppression). In Mindell's perspective, self-awareness begins with honest self-examination leading to acceptance not only of one's preferred identity but also the underlying less acceptable feelings such as anger, hatred, jealousy, vengeance, or greed.

It is possible that these underlying psycho-dynamics are themselves the outcomes of oppression that the involved individuals experience. In the last century Sennett and Cobb (1972) and Newby (1977) illustrated how the dynamics of social and economic class differences created internalized forms of oppression, in which people became deferential and powerless to those in authority, or assumed negative valuations of themselves; a good analogy is the movie *Titanic* in which third class passengers on the ship apparently accepted the precedence of first and second class passengers in evacuation (Lord, 1958). Gomberg (2007) explores similar concerns in the racial differences in contemporary America, and calls for a contributive justice based on opportunities that can confer social esteem. Forms of ill treatment are one of the tools of oppression, where the oppressed are treated so badly that they become convinced that they are inferior and unworthy, a dynamic that was very well described by Bettelheim (1970) and Frankl (1997). Both their narratives describe how some concentration camp prisoners simply gave up the battle to survive and ultimately died. This treatment may also lead to self-hatred as Frantz Fanon (1986) suggested. It is perhaps this self-hatred that leads to the presumed liberators becoming oppressive to the very people they sought to liberate, who look like them and therefore reflect to them the internal feelings of self-hatred. Such dictators use torture, which is part of the recipe for oppression and is intended to, as Black (2011, p. 219) observed, fuel 'a cycle of intimidation, alienation, ultimately corrupting human connections and creating isolation'. The internal personal dynamics resulting from the experience of oppression have to be examined honestly if the cycle that Black spoke about is to be broken.

Only when those intra-psychic aspects of self are expressed can there be true personal transformation. In this regard, Mindell stated: 'No vision or government can succeed unless we are aware of fear, rank, oppression, power and abuse by outer and internalized officials' (1995, p. 177). While Mindell was here speaking about social change, the same can be said of individuals and their relationships with the context in which they exist. One cannot have a clear, authentic, and enduring vision of his life without an awareness of the internalized fear, self-oppression, powerlessness, and internalized doubts that interfere with attempts to self-actualize. At this point, we suggest that you try to help your client increase self-awareness by completing the following exercise. Students (and therapists) can apply all the exercises in this chapter to themselves as part of experiential learning, to help them gain insights that may help them be better guides to their clients. The exercise below is an adaptation of the one proposed by Mindell (1995, p. 177). To clarify one's values broadly (consistent with the belief establishment phase of the IOT model) as part of the self-awareness development effort, we adopt Mindell's suggestion that a person ask him/herself the following questions:

1. *What kind of organizations do you prefer to support?*
   Think about one of these organizations.' An organization that you support could be a church (or other type of religious organization), a charity, a support group, a political party, a social club, etc.

2. *What vision does this group profess?*
   How is this vision consistent with your view of yourself, other people, society, and the environment? How is the vision inconsistent with your view of yourself, other people, society, or the environment?

3. *Who are the real or imagined opponents of your group?*
   [This helps the individual identify the stakeholders in the values represented by an organization that one supports, which by extension can be seen as that person's values] What kinds of belief systems or views is this group trying to overcome in the community in order to achieve its goals? How does your group deal or try to deal with those belief systems? How consistent is your group's plans to overcome opposing views with your own beliefs and values? If the group's plans and actions are not in agreement with your own beliefs and value system, why do you continue to support it?

Guide your client in reflecting carefully on the above questions and writing down her answers in as much detail as possible. Again, the above reflection is designed to help clients increase understanding of their personal motivations, hopefully leading to transformation of perspectives about themselves, other people, and the world. While considering the questions above, it is important to remember that patterns of social participation in organizations are changing due to complex factors interacting in society such as reduced access to opportunities, changing work patterns, available resources, and cultural influences. However, human beings continue to be inherently social (Marsh et al., 2007; Thieme et al., 2012). The social identities which are associated with belonging to social groups and organizations are important to human well-being (Hogg, 2001; Stets & Burke, 2000). According to the social identity theory, a social group 'creates and defines an individual's own place in society' (Tajfel, 1972, p. 293) because it provides roles for individual members which come with expectations and shared meanings. That is why social groups to which individuals belong are probably an expression of their own values, which are the basis of their social identity.

Consider an individual such as a student who belongs to a chapter of a professional association on campus. Members of such a group may be expected to volunteer for 'meals on wheels' in order to provide food to invalid older adults in the community, organize sessions to educate the community about the profession, raise money to help organizational members attend a professional conference, and so on. Such activities may be seen as being consistent with the individual's beliefs and values since the person chooses to be in the social group voluntarily. By completing such tasks, the individual experiences not only a sense of belonging but also enhanced self-esteem and sense of competency (Hornsey, 2008; Stets & Burke, 2000), and a transformation of self-conception and assimilation of 'all aspects of one's attitudes, feelings, and behaviors to the ingroup prototype' which changes how a person thinks, feels, and acts (Hogg, 2001, p. 187). Social identity theory suggests that belonging to social groups is very important for a meaningful life, not only because it is a way of achieving self-transcendence in Frankl's sense, but because such groups meet a fundamental need for human beings. Research shows that even though social identity in the 21st century has shifted away from identification with class, race, and nationality, people still seek to belong to groups, even though such groups are defined in new ways. In one study, Marsh et al. (2007) found that:

> Instead of thinking about belonging in terms of one group, or one specific place, it is now far more common for people to incorporate multiple social identities or a sense of belonging to a number of different groups and places at any one time in the course of their lives. Only 14% of poll participants agreed that they felt a strong sense of belonging to one particular social group, as opposed to 34% who said that their sense of belonging had changed significantly during the course of their lives. One aspect of this transition, then, is greater social freedom — we are able to join and leave certain social groups more easily than in the past. (p. 10

After the reflection guided by the exercise presented above, to increase self-understanding even further, administer the Appraisal of Perception of Meaning in Life (APML) introduced in chapter one (p. 69) to the client. You may also administer other validated instruments such as the Life Attitude Profile (LAP) assessment (Reker, n.d). These assessments can help clients further understand their sense of purposefulness in life, before you begin planning change initiatives in collaboration with them. Once the self-understanding has occurred, development of the personal mission in life can begin. To help the client articulate a personal mission statement, please use the guided imagery on page one of the Assessment and Intervention Instrument for Instrumentalism in Occupational Therapy (AIIIOT, see Appendix).

The term mission statement is not to be understood as the banal expression of a corporate identity. In this book, a personal mission is viewed as a compass to orient the individual in life, so that one is not lost in it. To borrow the alpinist metaphor from Frankl (1969), think of yourself as being in a forest, heading to a cabin that you know is there and will provide you with shelter and safety. However, you are surrounded by thick fog and cannot see your way to the destination. You begin to panic because you might get lost and die in the forest. The panic results in severe exhaustion and you almost give up. However, miraculously, the fog clears, and now you can clearly discern the cabin in the distance. This clearance of the fog gives you power and vitality. Suddenly, all the exhaustion is gone and you are re-motivated to continue on your journey. The stated mission should clear the fog in the forest of the client's life so that the legacy that he/she wants to create in the world is discernible in the distance, thus empowering him/her to continue more sure-footedly on the journey.

As mentioned earlier, the personal mission statement encompasses an individual's entire life including family, peer relationships, work, and community participation, and therefore covers the six dimensions of positive human health as identified by Hasselkus (2002, p. 61): 'self-acceptance, positive relations with others, autonomy, environmental mastery, purpose in life, and personal growth'. A principled life based on such a personal mission is also consistent with the three sources of meaning (establishment of emotionally intense *relationships*, participation in enjoyable and meaningful *work and leisure activities*, and adherence to *idea systems* [connecting to a larger reality than oneself, where this reality is the reality of transcendent ideas]); and the four dimensions of meaning (sense of *self-worth*, the sense that one has a *purpose in life*, sense of *control* in one's life circumstances, and ability to express one's *values*) as discussed in chapter 4. If clients live in a way that is consistent with the visualized mission in life, they would be working towards goals that they perceive to be worthwhile and in that way they would be likely to optimize their meaning in life as proposed by Frankl (1992). It should however be born in mind that the work with clients should always be client-centred. Therefore, the worth of the goals is determined by the client's social and cultural context rather than the practitioner's preferences.

Case example: Tammy

The following case example illustrates how to apply the guidelines discussed in this chapter. Tammy (not her real name), was a participant in a research study (see Ikiugu, Anderson, & Manas, 2008) which was designed to test the reliability of the Assessment and Intervention Instrument for Instrumentalism in Occupational Therapy [AIIIOT] (Ikiugu, 2007, 2004c). She came from the USA 'Bible Belt' (which includes largely the mid-West and Southern parts of the nation), where people are largely religious and conservative, and the issues she identified in her mission statement should be viewed against this geopolitical context.

This case illustrates the argument that while using the IOT as a guide to intervention, the practitioner's role is not to tell people how to approach life, or what kind of goals to strive for, even when some of the goals towards which the client works may present challenges to the perspectives of the practitioner. For example, a more liberal therapist with feminist leanings may consider Tammy's gaols to be too religious in nature, or Tammy as too much of a 'goody-two-shoes' kind of character. However, it is not in the place of the therapist using a client-centred perspective to dictate to Tammy what goals she should pursue, unless through therapy, Tammy somehow gains insight and desires to change her perspective. In other words, the role of the practitioner is merely to be a facilitator to the client's process. As Mindell (1985) once suggested, the role of the therapist is analogous to that of a mid-wife, who does not make babies but merely delivers them. Using the IOT provides an opportunity to educate people and to help them give birth to awareness of ideas that guide their decisions about what they do and why they do it.

Bearing in mind the above introduction explaining the role of the therapist/practitioner, following is Tammy's case. Based on guidance by the therapist using the AIIIOT protocol, Tammy wrote the following mission statement:

Tammy's visualized perception of self by others. Tammy was a student on a two year, 80 credit program leading to a Master of Science degree in occupational therapy. It was a very rigorous program of study, and caused students much stress. Many of them felt as if their lives were out of balance. Tammy identified herself as a devout Christian who tried to observe the teachings of her faith, including being self-less in her service to her husband-to-be, family, and other people. These dictates of her faith tended to present problems because of the need to balance them with a demanding degree program. Tammy felt that she did not have much time for socialization and it was a challenge even to find time to spend with loved ones (such as her fiancé). She found it a challenge to find time every evening to call her fiancé although she knew it was important for the health of their developing relationship to communicate with him regularly. With a holiday approaching she felt that she needed some time for herself when she could forget the demands on her time at least for a while. With these issues in mind, Tammy imagined significant people in her life making the following statements about her:

A. **Family member:**
I appreciate all she does. She works hard in school and then always drives to see me. She needed this vacation.

B. **Social Life (friend):**
We don't get to see Tammy very often because she is so busy all the time. We are looking forward to spending more time with her.

C. **Work/professional colleague:**
Tammy works for us every weekend to help pay for the wedding. We appreciate her loyalty to us. She deserves this break.

D. **Church/community organization member:**
We are so excited to have Tammy as a member of our church. I feel she will be a great asset to us. We just want to make sure her spiritual life comes first, before her busy-ness.

Tammy's mission statement

Based on these imagined statements, Tammy articulated her mission statement as follows: 'My mission in life is to center all aspects of my life on God's everyday will for me by loving and being a support for my family, showing my care and compassion for friends, by being dedicated to integrity and justice in my profession and professional development, and by continuing to participate in community activities for the development of the community as well as myself'.

Action

Choosing occupations to help create desired legacy

Once the mission statement is articulated, go to section II of the AIIIOT. In the spaces provided under each of the four categories of the mission statement (family, social life, work/professional life, and affiliation to community organization(s), ask your client to list up to two occupations which if performed adequately and with the desired frequency, would help him achieve his mission in life. Tammy listed the following as the occupations that she thought would help her achieve her personal mission:

Family

1. Speaking with her fiancé on the phone every day
2. Visiting family regularly together with fiancé

Social life

1. Visiting with a friend
2. Speaking with friends who live far away over the phone

Work/professional life

1. Completing her professional development assessment
2. Keeping a planner and completing all the activities on the planner (i.e. developing an action plan with delineated tasks and times for their completion)

Affiliation to church/community organization(s)

1. Regularly attending church and church activities
2. Becoming active in a church program, for example, a care group

Self-rating on performance and satisfaction with performance of chosen occupations

Once clients have identified occupations that would help them achieve the stated life mission, ask them to rate themselves on the four scales of the AIIIOT (section III of the AIIIOT). For example, Tammy rated herself as shown in Table 6.1 overleaf:

Table 6.1
Tammy's Self-Rating on Occupations identified as Important for Achievement of her Personal Mission in Life

Area of Mission Statement	Frequency	Adequacy	Satisfaction	Belief
Speaking with fiancé on the phone every day	3	3	3	3
Visiting family regularly together with fiancé	2	3	2	3
Visiting with a friend	3	3	2	3
Speaking with friends who live far away over the phone	2	3	1	3
Completing professional development assessment	1	1	1	3
Keeping a current planner and completing activities on the planner	3	3	2	3
Regularly attending church and church activities	3	3	3	4
Becoming active in a church program, for example, a care group	1	1	1	3
Total	**18**	**20**	**15**	**25**
Index (raw score/number of listed occupations=8)	**2.25**	**2.5**	**1.88**	**3.13**

Planning action to create change

The whole purpose of the ensuing exercises (increasing self-awareness and assessment) is to create change so as to maximize meaning in one's life through daily occupational performance. An important step in this process is to establish goals that would ensure that this change is achieved. The goals should be Relevant, specify how long it will take to achieve them, Understandable, Measurable, Behavioral, and Achievable [RHUMBA] (Sames, 2014). In formulating goals, performance of occupations on which the client's self-rating of satisfaction with performance is less than 4 are targeted for improvement. This is because if the client is satisfied with performance of an occupation, even if such performance is not optimum, there is no need to try to change it. Consistent with the client-centered perspective of the IOT model, the practitioner only needs to help the client change performance of occupations with which he/she is not satisfied. Tammy developed seven goals to optimize performance of the seven occupations on which she rated herself less than 4 in satisfaction:

Short-term goals

1. Within two weeks, I will have improved my interaction with my fiancé as indicated by speaking with him on the phone at least once a day, 7 days a week.
2. Within four weeks, I will demonstrate improved participation in family-oriented activities as indicated by visiting both my family and my fiance's family with him at least once a week.
3. In 3 weeks, my social life will have improved significantly as indicated by visiting with a friend for at least one hour once a week.
4. Within 4 weeks, my social life will have improved significantly as indicated by speaking with a friend on the phone at least twice a week.
5. In two weeks, I will have made significant progress towards achieving my professional career goals as indicated by completing my professional development assessment and clearly identifying the skills I need to develop for success in my future career.
6. In five weeks, I will have made significant progress towards achieving my professional goals as indicated by keeping a daily planner with professional activities to help me develop the skills I need and completing each activity on the planner at least once/week.
7. Within 4 weeks, I will demonstrate increased participation in church activities as indicated by participating in a church care group at least twice per week.

Long-term goals

Within one year, I will have made significant progress towards my stated mission as indicated by a satisfaction self-rating of 4/4 in at least 4 out of the 8 occupations that I listed on the AIIIOT during this assessment.

No plan for change results in any tangible consequences unless it is actually acted upon. Therefore, the next step in creating change to optimize meaning in life is for the client to commit to action according to established goals. Such action may include: improving skills (e.g., Tammy may decide to attend a workshop in which she can learn the professional skills that she needs as identified in the professional development assessment [goal # 6]); developing new routines that are consistent with the desired outcomes (e.g. establishing a weekly routine to ensure that engagement in the activities in the established planner become habitual [goal # 7]), etc.

Consequence appraisal

The construct of historicity in the philosophy of pragmatism refers to the idea that the present emerges from experiences in the past and then extends to an imagined future. This imagining thus creates a continuity of experience from the past, present, and future (Mead, 1932). According to Mead, the continuity that allows past experiences to contribute to emergence of desired consequences is what has made the human being so successful in adapting to the environment. This view is consistent with the idea in narrative psychology that: 'All other things being equal, a life story that explains clearly how a person came to be who he or she is – a narrative that integrates a life in time – is 'better' than one that does not' (McAdams, 2006, p. 117). Consistent with this construct of historicity, one of the basic premises in the Instrumentalism in Occupational Therapy (IOT) theoretical conceptual practice model is that effective use of the mind denotes the ability to learn from the past and use this learning to modify current behavior in order to achieve desired outcomes in the future (Ikiugu, 2004a). As McAdams (2006) would put it, effective use of the mind denotes the ability to 'reconstruct the past and anticipate the future in such a way as to provide life with identity, meaning, and coherence' (pp. 109-110).

In other words, an individual first acts in accordance with current beliefs that are based in past experiences, and examines the consequences of the action in order to determine whether the outcome is as expected (confirmation of beliefs according to Peirce, 1955). If the consequences are as expected, the belief is confirmed, the action is deemed to be adaptive, and it continues into the future, and one's life course is experienced as having coherence and meaning. If the consequences are different from what was expected, the individual is in a state of doubt, which leads to examination of the beliefs on which the action was based, leading to development of new beliefs (in the form of new hypotheses, or in case of IOT, revision of one's perceived mission in life) or thinking of new occupations or adjusting actions to help achieve the existing beliefs (or mission in life in terms of IOT terminology). Ikiugu (2004a, 2004b, 2004c) referred to this process as the consequence appraisal phase of the IOT.

When working with clients', the practitioner should set aside time for re-assessment as they commit to action in pursuit of established goals (re-assessment could be set in weekly or bi-weekly periods). At these pre-established re-assessment times, the AIIIOT is re-administered. At each re-assessment, previous AIIIOT scores are subtracted from the current ones in order to determine whether progress has been made towards established goals. If progress on any of the goals is not being made, the clients' mission statements and/or the occupations that were chosen to help them achieve the mission are re-examined, and in collaboration with the practitioner, the mission statement may be changed, or occupations and planned action strategies may be adjusted. In the example given earlier, Tammy was not re-assessed because she was involved in an instrument validation study rather than an intervention. An example from a recent study will serve to illustrate how scores can be used to indicate progress towards identified goals or lack thereof.

Case study: Greg

In this study, the effectiveness of the Modified Instrumentalism in Occupational Therapy (MIOT theoretical model) in facilitating change in occupational behavior among the study participants so that their occupational performance was more consistent with amelioration of global issues of concern to humankind such as climate change was tested (Ikiugu, Cerny, Nissen et al., in press). The sample consisted of 6 participants, two men and four women. Three of the participants were graduate occupational therapy students, all women, ages 22 to 24 years. The other three participants were faculty members at the University of South Dakota and ranged in age from mid-30s to mid-60s. The participant described below (Greg, not his real name) was a faculty member, male, in his mid-30s. At pretest, he wrote his mission statement as follows:

Greg's visualized perception of self by others at pretest

Family member
Greg is concerned about poverty, especially as it is the product of unfettered capitalism. He strongly believes/feels that everyone should have enough to eat, medical care, and access to education. He is concerned about diseases that harm people but for which treatment exists and is not available. Greg likes fuel-efficient cars and espouses the development of better, efficient rail/public transportation system in the US.

Friend
Greg is concerned but not very vocal about how he feels about these things. He is very open-minded and tolerant of ambiguity.

Colleague
I have little knowledge of Greg's stance on social issues, except the more Universal (socialization) of educational opportunity.

Community Organization
I have no idea about Greg's sense of these issues. He does like local foods and sustainable agriculture due to his participation in the V area Farmer's market.

Greg's pretest mission statement

My mission in life is to:

1. Be a good father
2. Be a good husband
3. Be a good friend, colleague, and statistician
4. Learn and explore thoughts, ideas, skills, and art. Be open to anything
5. Get better at those things that are:
   a. Good to do
   b. I am good at doing
   c. I want to do

Greg listed the following occupations as appropriate to help him achieve the above-stated mission:

Family
1. Playing with and reading to the daughter
2. Telling wife that he loves her

Social life
1. Working with the community guild
2. Forming a sculling club

Work
1. Learning Bayesian statistics better
2. Writing a grant

Community participation
1. Being more helpful at the local farmer's market
2. Hosting a woodwork class

Greg rated himself on the AIIIOT as shown in Table 6.2 overleaf.

Greg's goal was to improve his frequency and adequacy of performance of occupations on which he rated himself less than 4 on satisfaction (basically all the 8 identified occupations). At posttest, he wrote his personal mission statement as follows:

Table 6.2
Greg's Self-Rating on Occupations identified as Important for Achievement of his Personal Mission in Life at Pretest

Area of Mission Statement	Frequency	Adequacy	Satisfaction	Belief
Playing with/reading to daughter	3	3	2	4
Telling wife he loves her	3	3	3	4
Working with the local community guild	2	2	1	3
Forming a sculling club	1	2	1	2
Learning Bayesian Statistics better	4	3	3	4
Writing another grant	2	3	3	3
Helping at the local farmer's market	2	3	2	3
Hosting a woodworking class	1	3	1	3
Total	**18**	**22**	**16**	**26**
Index (raw score/number of listed occupations=8)	**2.25**	**2.75**	**2.0**	**3.25**

Greg's visualized perception of self by others at posttest

Family Member

Daughter - Daddy plays with me, tickles me, and gives me candy. Wife - Greg can be aloof, withdrawn, and difficult to engage at times, but I know he loves me. He gives of himself to organizations that need help, but seems to do so in an idiosyncratic manner.

Friend

Greg and I enjoy great laughs and go to one another when we are having problems in our lives. He always gives me good advice. He keeps his world views close to his vest most of the time.

Colleague

Greg is a very knowledgeable and helpful statistician. I have little idea about his sense of global issues.

Community Member

Greg has been busy lately with work and family. He has not been as active as he was a few years ago. He seems to like conserving forest products and energy as part of his woodworking hobby.

Greg's posttest mission statement

> My mission in life is to be the best father and husband that I can be. Second to that, I want to be a good friend and colleague when/where I can be. Finally, I want to pursue my love of rowing and woodworking. To these ends, I can continue to conserve and help keep the world viable for humans, including, especially, my daughter.

Gregg identified the following occupations as relevant in helping him achieve the above-stated mission:

Family
1. Playing with and reading to the daughter
2. Setting aside 'spouse time'

Social life
1. Spending more time woodworking with friends
2. Having couples' nights out

Work
1. Finding ways of improving students' understanding of statistics
2. Helping people make better decisions based on statistics

Community participation
1. Establishing a rowing club
2. Helping at the farmer's market

At posttest, Greg rated himself on the AIIIOT as shown in table 6.3 overleaf.

Greg's change in self-rating (indicating progress towards his personal mission statement) was: frequency of engagement in occupations that are important for achievement of mission=2.63-2.25=.38; perceived adequacy of performance of occupations perceived to be important in achieving personal mission=3.25-2.75=.50; satisfaction with performance=2.88-2.0=.88; and belief in ability to perform identified occupations=3.88-3.25=.63. Thus, Greg made progress in all areas of his mission statement and therefore, it can be assumed that he perceived himself as progressing towards his personal mission in life, and to that extent, he experienced his life as increasingly purposeful and meaningful.

The reader should notice a few things from the above example: First, as you work with a client, her mission statement can change over time as she gains more insight into her life circumstances. Secondly, what are important are not the specific occupations that are identified as being important for achievement of mission in life. Rather, what is important is the self-rating on the four AIIIOT scales in respect to the chosen occupations. Thus, at retest, the occupations that are seen as important for achievement of personal mission can change. However,

Table 6.3
Greg's Self-Rating on Occupations identified as Important for Achievement of his Personal Mission in Life at Posttest

Area of Mission Statement	Frequency	Adequacy	Satisfaction	Belief
Playing with/reading to daughter	3	3	2.5	4
Setting aside "spouse time"	2	3	2.5	3
Spending more time woodworking with friends	2	3	2	4
Having couples' nights out	1	3	3	4
Finding ways of improving students' understanding of statistics	4	3.5	3	4
Helping people make better decisions based on statistics	4	3.5	3	4
Establishing a rowing club	2	3	4	4
Helping at the farmer's market	3	4	3	4
Total	**21**	**26**	**23**	**31**
Index (raw score/number of listed occupations=8)	**2.63**	**3.25**	**2.88**	**3.88**

the self-rating on the four scales is still able to indicate whether progress is being made towards the established mission. In addition to the weekly or biweekly re-assessment as described above, after a reasonable length of time (e.g. 5 weeks), another assessment such as the Life Attitude Profile (LAP) can be re-administered to determine the extent to which the client's sense of purpose and meaning in life has changed. Now, help your client articulate a mission statement, identify occupations to actualize that mission, rate himself on the four AIIIOT scales, and develop a plan to improve performance and satisfaction with performance of those occupations.

General comments about the Proposed Change Protocol

The reader might have noticed that the IOT/MIOT-based process embraces both cognitive and behavioral intervention strategies. The individual who wants to create change visualizes not only the desired change but also the view of oneself as an agent of change, as well as how other people and the environment in general affect or fit into the process of change. This approach is consistent with the available research evidence which clearly indicates the clinical effectiveness of Cognitive Behavioral therapeutic strategies. It has been found that use of Cognitive Behavioral Therapy (CBT) as a guide to intervention is associated with increased remission of psychotic symptoms among individuals with mental illness, decreased panic episodes among those with panic disorders, decreased anxiety and depression, etc. (Addis et al., 2006; Cavanagh et al., 2006; Lewis et al., 2002). In occupational therapy, cognitive behavioral strategies have been found to be moderately effective in improving engagement in physical activities and long-term exercise routines among community-dwelling older adults (Arbesman & Mosley, 2012). Therefore, using the IOT/MIOT principles to guide occupational performance change in order to optimize meaning in life would be consistent with the best available evidence since it is a very cognitive/behavioral process. Available evidence supports the effectiveness of such guidelines (cognitive-behavioral strategies) in creating behavioral change.

Secondly, the IOT/MIOT principles guide interventions designed to create total lifestyle change that incorporates all aspects of a person's life (family, socialization, work, and community participation). This approach requires complete overhaul of one's habits and routines consistent with the pragmatic principle of the importance of habits in supporting adaptive behavior as articulated by James (1981). James was of the opinion that habits are so important that they support adaptive functioning not only for individuals but also for entire societies. We are able to function as a society, he argued, only because we have established habits that help us anticipate the outcome of our actions, what to expect from other people, etc. According to James, people who want to change their lives must change their actions which in turn will result in a change of consequences. This change cannot be done piece-meal. It must constitute a complete overhaul of one's lifestyle. This is the same idea in complexity theory, that in order to change the system trajectory, perturbation (energy, for example in form of information) must be introduced (Ikiugu, 2007, 2005; Ikiugu & Rosso, 2005). The perturbation in turn leads to reorganization of the entire system (something akin to lifestyle re-design) and subsequent change in the system trajectory.

For example, smokers who want to simply abstain from smoking may find it very challenging to do so without adopting an entire non-smoking lifestyle.

Adopting a non-smoking lifestyle would mean not frequenting places where smoking tends to happen (such as bars), avoiding some routines that in the past have been associated with smoking, and sometimes even avoiding friends who used to be smoking buddies for a while (at least until the non-smoking lifestyle is firmly established). The idea that habits are at the core of lifestyle change was later used by Slagle in her famous habit training programs in the early 20th century occupational therapy (Bockoven, 1971; Ikiugu, 2007), and has persisted as an important aspect of the habituation component of the human system as described by Kielhofner (2008) in the Model of Human Occupation (MOHO). Further, lifestyle overhaul characterized by making changes in occupational habits and routines consistent with healthy living, is an important element of the Lifestyle Redesign program developed by researchers at the University of Southern California (Jackson et al., 1998). Lifestyle Redesign facilitates individual recognition of self as an occupational being. Research evidence suggests that the program is effective in improving the sense of well-being and quality of life among community-dwelling older adults (Clark et al., 2011).

This evidence supports the value of protocols such as the one based on the IOT/MIOT principles described in this chapter in creating the desired change to enhance a sense of meaning in life, and by extension quality of life through carefully designed occupational performance routines. The IOT/MIOT-based protocol satisfies all the criteria for effective life change interventions as identified in recent systematic reviews of evidence supporting the clinical effectiveness of occupational therapy interventions (Arbesman & Mosley, 2012), which indicates that:

> ...effectiveness appears to be higher for client-centered programs that are tailored to the program participant...individualization of self-management programs includes providing health-related information to the client, *reflecting on available options, and then developing a program according to the client's preferences*. (p. 280, emphasis added)

Clearly, the IOT/MIOT-based guidelines provide a client-centered approach in which the partner in the intervention is helped through the process of: self-exploration, which increases self-awareness (acquisition of information about self); reflection on options available for lifestyle change (through development of a personal mission statement and identification of occupations to help clients achieve the mission); and development of a plan of action to help them achieve the goals that help them make progress towards the personal mission in life.

Conclusion

In the first 5 chapters of this book, we discussed various aspects of meaning-making through daily occupational performance. In this chapter we introduced a theoretical conceptual practice model, Instrumentalism in Occupational Therapy (IOT)/Modified Instrumentalism in Occupational Therapy (MIOT), as a 'how to' conceptual framework to guide occupational behavior change. The process begins with reflection exercises to help the client increase self-awareness. Based on this increased self-awareness, the client is guided through establishment of a personal mission statement to act as a compass to direct her towards what is purposeful and meaningful in life. Occupations are chosen that are visualized as important in helping her actualize the stated mission in life, and self-assessment on the frequency, adequacy, belief, and satisfaction with performance of the identified occupations is administered. Goals are established targeting improvement of performance of occupations on whose rating of satisfaction with performance is less than optimal. The person commits to actions geared towards improvement of those occupations and self-assessment and adjustment of the action plan are done regularly until established goals are achieved. This approach enhances creative use of personal talents, self-transcendence, and connection to other people leading to a sense of meaning in life as conceptualized by Frankl (1992).

Appendix

Assessment and Intervention Instrument for Instrumentalism in Occupational Therapy (AIIOT)

When using this instrument, the therapist should find a quiet place where the client can concentrate and respond in detail to all items without interruption. The client should be given as much time as necessary to respond to all items in this instrument exhaustively. The instrument consists of four sections. In section I, a personal mission statement is created. This provides a purpose towards which the client strives. In section II, occupations in whose regular engagement would lead to achievement of the stated mission in life are identified. In section III, the client's self-perception of engagement in identified occupations is rated on four scales: frequency, adequacy, satisfaction, and belief in ability to engage in the occupations. In section IV, the self-rating scores are added together to give engagement indexes on the four scales.

I. Personal Mission Statement

The therapist should read the following directions loudly to guide the client in completing this exercise (see Covey, 1990).

Imagine that one day, you come home unexpectedly. You find a large group of people meeting in the house. As you come in, you find that for some reason, they are all talking about you. You decide to listen to what they are saying. No one knows you are there. Write down in detail what you would like to hear each of the following say about you: (a) family member (father, mother, spouse, son/daughter, sister/brother, cousin, any other family member that you feel close to). (b) Friends (one or two close friends). (c) work/professional colleague/associate. (d) a member of the church or some other community organization to which you are affiliated. Now, go over what you have written down and take a few moments to think about what you imagine each of those people saying about you. These statements represent the kind of person you would like to be and that you can be. Summarize the statements in a few sentences, stating what you consider to be your personal mission statement. This mission statement will provide the direction towards which you will strive from now on. The statement should consist of four components corresponding to the four areas of the overheard conversations: family, friends, work/professional life, and engagement in Church/community organization(s).

II. Identification of Occupations

For each of the four areas, identify two occupations in whose regular engagement will lead to achievement of the stated mission in life.

A. Family

1.____

2.____

B. Social Life (Friendship)

1.____

2.____

C. Work/Professional Life

1.____

2.____

D. Affiliation to Church/Community Organization(s)

1.____

2.____

III. Evaluation

For each of the identified occupations, rate yourself on a scale from one (1) to four (4) regarding: (a) frequency, (b) adequacy, (c) satisfaction, and (d) belief about your ability to engage in the occupation.

Descriptors

Frequency

1 = do not engage in the occupation; 2 = rarely engages in the occupation; 3 = regularly engages in the occupation; 4 = frequently engages in the occupation as necessary.

Adequacy

1 = I am not able to engage in the occupation; 2 = I engage in the occupation with difficulty and the outcome is inadequate; 3 = I engage in the occupation with difficulty but the outcome is good when able to complete it; 4 = I engage in the occupation, am able to complete it, and the outcome is always adequate.

Satisfaction

1= I am disappointed with my engagement in the occupation; 2 = I am somewhat satisfied with my engagement in the occupation; 3 = I am satisfied with my engagement in the occupation but would like to improve; 4 = I am happy with my engagement in the occupation as it is.

Belief

1 = I do not believe that I am capable of engaging in this occupation; 2 = I believe that I can engage in the occupation with much help; 3 = I believe I can engage in the occupation with a little help; 4 = I believe I can engage in the occupation independently with desired frequency and adequacy.

	Frequency	Adequacy	Satisfaction	Belief
	1 2 3 4	1 2 3 4	1 2 3 4	1 2 3 4
A. Family				
1.	___ ___ ___ ___	___ ___ ___ ___	___ ___ ___ ___	___ ___ ___ ___
2.	___ ___ ___ ___	___ ___ ___ ___	___ ___ ___ ___	___ ___ ___ ___
B. Social Life (Friendship)				
1.	___ ___ ___ ___	___ ___ ___ ___	___ ___ ___ ___	___ ___ ___ ___
2.	___ ___ ___ ___	___ ___ ___ ___	___ ___ ___ ___	___ ___ ___ ___
C. Work/Professional Life				
1.	___ ___ ___ ___	___ ___ ___ ___	___ ___ ___ ___	___ ___ ___ ___
2.	___ ___ ___ ___	___ ___ ___ ___	___ ___ ___ ___	___ ___ ___ ___
D. Affiliation to Church/Community Organization(s)				
1.	___ ___ ___ ___	___ ___ ___ ___	___ ___ ___ ___	___ ___ ___ ___
2.	___ ___ ___ ___	___ ___ ___ ___	___ ___ ___ ___	___ ___ ___ ___
Scores (x11, x12, x13, x14)	________	________	________	________
	Frequency	Adequacy	Satisfaction	Belief
Scale Index=Total/# of occupations	________	________	________	________

To obtain aggregate scores for each of the four scales, add together the ratings in each column and place the total at the bottom of the column. These scores are denoted x11, x12, x13, and x14 for frequency, adequacy, satisfaction, and belief respectively. To obtain an index for each scale, divide the aggregate score by the number of listed occupations. The index should be between one and four. During re-assessment, the client should rate him/herself on the four scales again, the scores aggregated as before, and divided by the number of listed occupations. If the client changes the occupations that he/she perceives to lead to achievement of personal mission in life, use a new AIIIOT form to rate the client on the four scales. The sum of self-ratings, however, should be denoted x21, x22, x23, and x24 respectively in either case. Progress in therapy is indicated by; x21-x11, x22-x12, x23-x13, and x24-x14 respectively.

Comments:

PART IV
OCCUPATIONAL THERAPY, OCCUPATIONAL SCIENCE, AND FUTURE OCCUPATIONAL NEEDS

In the final part of the book, we discuss our thoughts about a possible future of occupational therapy and occupational science given the ideas that we proposed in the preceding chapters. We suggest that occupational therapy and occupational science could be a premier profession and scientific discipline by heeding the call as articulated in the American Occupational Therapy Association's (AOTA) centennial vision to meet society's occupational needs. We argue that perhaps the best way the profession of occupational therapy and the discipline of occupational science can serve society in the future is by providing interventions and scholarly investigations geared towards meeting peoples' need for meaningful existence through occupational performance, in line with ideas about meaningful living through occupational performance as discussed in this book. Such service would require that occupational therapists and occupational scientists find ways of working with people in their communities, either individually or in groups, to address pertinent societal issues that threaten human survival by changing the way they choose and engage in daily occupations. We think that the thoughts presented in this section are an apt way to conclude the book and hope that the ideas that we have laid out will stimulate some debate about the direction that occupational therapy and occupational science could take in the future in order to serve society in the best way possible.

Chapter 7
Occupational therapy, occupational science and future occupational needs

Learning objectives

By the end of this chapter, the reader will be able to demonstrate an understanding of:

1. How meaning in life relates to a concern for all life on earth and for ensuring survival of humanity in the future
2. A possible broadened future role of occupational therapists and occupational scientists in joining other professional and scientific disciplines that are interested in working with individuals, small groups, and communities to resolve some of the issues of concern to humanity in general

Contents of this chapter

- The future of occupational therapy and occupational science: Realizing the objective of truly meeting society's occupational needs by helping people optimize meaning in their lives
  - Major issues of concern in contemporary society, and the potential of occupation-based solutions to those issues as a way of helping people relate to causes bigger than themselves and therefore optimize meaning in life
  - Harnessing human agency through occupational performance by working with individuals and communities as a way of shaping a promising future for humanity

Introduction

From time to time, professional organizations engage in reflection and self-examination to take stock of their achievements and to chart the way to the future. In the USA, the American Occupational Therapy Association (AOTA) began the celebration of a hundred years of the profession by specifying the goals to be met by the time of the centennary in 2017. The vision was stated as follows: "We envision that occupational therapy is a powerful, widely recognized, science-driven, and evidence-based profession with a globally connected and diverse workforce meeting society's occupational needs" (AOTA, 2006, p. 1). This is indeed a laudable vision. The question is: What are the society's occupational needs that the profession of occupational therapy should be striving to meet? How are occupational therapists and scientists going to meet those needs? In order to answer the above two questions, it is necessary to understand the social and ecological context in which the profession is currently operating to ascertain the society's occupational priorities and begin figuring out how to address them.

In this book, we began with the premise that one of the most important needs of our time is for people to engage in occupations that help them individually and collectively create meaning in their lives. Our focus in the previous six chapters was to examine and deepen an understanding of this need for meaning from multiple perspectives and to suggest ways of helping people use daily occupations to make their lives meaningful. As has been emphasized throughout the book, one of Frankl's (1992) propositions was that meaning results to a large extent from feeling a sense of connection to something larger than oneself. In order to help people connect to causes larger than themselves, occupational therapists and occupational scientists need to be cognizant of the wider social, historical, and environmental contexts. Having cognizance of these contexts could help us clarify and work towards realization of the full potential value of occupational therapy and occupational science to society.

In order to provide this clarification, in this chapter we will briefly examine the major issues of concern in contemporary society, and the potential role of occupational therapists and scientists in sensitizing people to help them actualize their agency in shaping a promising future for humanity, and in the process create ultimately meaningful existence in their own lives. We assume that when people resolve to commit to saving the life-supporting ecology of the earth, they contribute to the survival of posterity and there is no cause that is greater and therefore a source of more meaning than that.

Factors affecting future occupational justice in contemporary society

Population growth

The first major concern is that we have a rapidly growing population, with about 10,000 people being added into our planet every hour (Martin, 2011). According to the United Nations (UN) estimates, the current population is about 7 billion people. By the year 2050, we will be 9.3 billion strong, and 10.1 billion by the end of the century (UN, 2010). However, the actual population could vary from between 9.3 and 10.6 billion people by 2050 to between 10.1 and 15.8 billion people by 2100. These numbers are significant when considered within the historical context. It took about one million years for the population to grow to one billion people (Kelley, 1988). However, in the span of about 120 years, the number of people doubled to 2 billion, and in another 35 years, a third billion was added into the population. Between 1950 and 1990 (a span of 40 years), the population grew from 2.5 to 5 billion people (University of Michigan, 2006). These numbers have significant implications for the future of occupational therapy and occupational science. The rapidly growing population brings into question other issues of concern to occupational therapists and scientists such as environmental degradation, reduction of the earth's carrying capacity, and poverty. These issues affect the ability of human beings to access resources and to engage in meaningful occupations.

Environmental degradation

While it took one million years to reach a population of one billion people in 1800, in only 200 years, the population has increased sixfold (from one billion to about 7 billion). This rapid population growth poses a significant challenge. For each additional person on earth, we create a need for more food, water, and fuel to provide required energy (Daily & Ehrlich, 1992; Martin, 2011; Nassos, n.d.). Each additional person also contributes to accumulation of greenhouse gasses and other pollutants to the environment and therefore to the worsening problem of climate change. Considering that by estimates from many demographers (Daily & Ehrlich, 1992; Hardin, 1991; Woolley, 2009) we have already surpassed the carrying capacity of the earth, this rapid population growth, the ensuing demand for resources, and acceleration of pollution to the ecosystem has serious implications for the future survival of the human species.

Already, the environmental change due to a combination of increasing human population and unsustainable lifestyles has made many people in the world vulnerable. For example, a temperature rise by 1 degree Celsius has caused melting of the permafrost, decreasing ground water levels, and other problems leading to a decrease in availability of muskrats in the Peace Athabasca delta and other wild life in the Mackenzie basin in northeast Canada (Cohen et al., 1997). This decrease in wildlife to which the indigenous people in the region are dependent has reduced the human carrying capacity of the area threatening their survival. It has also affected these peoples' ability to engage in their traditional productive occupations, such as fishing to provide for their families. In the developed countries (most of them in the Northern hemisphere, but also in the southern regions of Latin America), there have been reports of record fatalities in recent years due to melanomas that can be attributed to depletion of the ozone layer. This is a result of human occupations that lead to accumulation of chlorofluorocarbons (CFCs) in the higher atmosphere resulting from use of refrigeration (United States Environmental Protection Agency [US EPA], 1998). Obviously, depletion of the protective ozone layer in the atmosphere reduces the earth's human carrying capacity overall.

An example from Africa includes the Lake Victoria basin in East Africa where the wetlands around the lake have been drained to give way to cultivation of rice, cotton, and sugar-cane to feed the increasing population (US EPA, 1998). Consequently, the natural filters to silt and plant nutrients in the soil have been destroyed leading to run-off of soil and the nutrients into the lake. This run-off has caused increased growth of algae that cloud the water surface, reducing oxygen concentration in the water and causing death of fish on which the people around the lake depend for survival (Fuggie, 2001). Overall, human activities that produce pollution "coupled with the rising population and mismanagement of available resources have caused environmental degradation and impacted negatively on the quality of life in the region" (Kiogora et al., 2011, p. 322).

These examples demonstrate how the exploding population growth is reducing the human carrying capacity and indeed threatening the survival of the human species into the future, in addition to impacting access to meaningful occupations by all human beings.

There are two types of carrying capacity: biophysical and social (Daily & Ehrlich, 1992; Woolley, 2009). According to ecological biologists, the biophysical carrying capacity refers to "the maximal population size of a given species that an area can support without reducing its ability to support the same species in the future" (Daily & Ehrlich, 1992, p. 3 of 19). This ability of an area to support current populations without jeopardizing future survival of the same species depends on the maximum sustainable use (MSU) of resources and the maximum sustainable abuse (MSA) of the eco-support systems. The MSU refers to the extent to which renewable resources such as forests and water can rejuvenate effectively after use, or can be substituted by other resources (such as replacement of wood fuel with natural gas for heating and cooking to avoid depletion of forest reserves). When use of renewable resources exceeds the MSU, the carrying capacity of a species is reduced, and survival of the species into the future is threatened. For example, depletion of forest reserves means that the natural carbon sink reservoir (forests absorb carbon dioxide and therefore prevent its accumulation into the atmosphere) is destroyed. This degradation of the carbon sink is related to acceleration of global warming and climate change which threatens viability of the human species on earth. Similarly, depletion of water aquifers means that human survival is compromised since there is no substitute for water, on which every living thing on earth is dependent.

The MSA refers to the extent to which the "biogeochemical processes to absorb waste and reconstitute component resources therein" (Daily & Ehrlich, 1992, p. 8 of 19) are not overwhelmed by overuse of resources and over production of waste due to human activities. When the capacity for the above mentioned biogeochemical processes to function effectively is exceeded, resources are depleted, the pollutants cannot be degraded fast enough so that they accumulate in the atmosphere, and the ability of the eco-system to support quality human life is compromised. This is already happening as indicated by the degradation of top-soil, water aquifers, forest cover, and accumulation of greenhouse gasses as discussed earlier. Essentially, the earth's human carrying capacity can be expressed in an equation as follows: $K=MSU+MSA$, where K=carrying capacity; MSU=maximum sustainable use of resources; and MSA=maximum sustainable abuse of the life-supporting eco-system.

Social carrying capacity refers to "lifestyle aspirations, epidemiological factors, patterns of socially controlled resource distribution, the disparity between private and social costs, the difficult in formulating rational policy in the face of uncertainty, and various other features of human sociopolitical and economic organization" (Daily & Ehrlich, 1992, p. 10 of 19) that interfere with the ability of humanity to live on earth in a sustainable manner. One can visualize the social carrying capacity as the lifestyle, demographic, and governance factors that lead to sustainability or unsustainability and therefore either to the maintenance or reduction of the earth's biophysical carrying capacity.

For example, continued over-reliance on fossil fuels and the inability of world governments to work on finding alternative sources of energy due to economic self-interest of fossil fuel-based corporations that wield much power over the governments leads to lifestyles that cause humanity to exceed MSA (by causing accumulation of greenhouse gasses at a rate that exceeds the natural carbon degradation process, and therefore causing climate change) and this subsequently leads to a decrease in the earth's carrying capacity. Similarly, public policies that do not encourage cognizance of the number of people on earth lead to unsustainable population growth. This causes depletion of both renewable and non-renewable resources and the degradation of the eco-support systems, subsequently leading to a reduction in the earth's biophysical carrying capacity for human beings. An example of the impact of reduction in biophysical and social carrying capacities is clear in the following statement by the United Nations Environmental Program [UNEP] (n.d., p. 306):

> ... water tables are falling fast under the North China plain. In 1997, almost 100,000 wells were abandoned apparently because they ran dry as the water table fell, but 221,900 new wells were drilled. The drilling of so many wells reflects a desperate quest for water.

For occupational therapy and occupational science, exceeding MSU and MSA due to population growth and unsustainable lifestyles means that human beings cannot effectively engage satisfactorily in occupations that sustain them (such as farming, fishing, hobbies). As Max-Neef (2010) argues, all these occupations constitute real needs that people have to meet not only in order to survive but also in order to enjoy themselves as human beings. Consequently their ability to live meaningful lives is compromised (for example, lack of water means that those who like to do gardening for leisure cannot do it as much as they like, and depletion of forests means that those who like working with wood do not have the resources to participate in this valuable leisure activity). To illustrate this point, when the first author was a child, one of the most enjoyable pastimes for his mother was making sisal baskets. This leisure occupation resulted in beautiful baskets that were used to carry produce and other things. She taught his sisters this skill, but because of climate change, sisal does not grow in the area any more. Therefore, his sisters cannot enjoy this leisure occupation that they learned from their mother. In other words, exceeding MSU and MSA threatens not only the physical survival of the human species, but also the ability to engage in everyday meaningful occupations. This leads to an overall decline in the human quality of life. These threats directly impact on the ability of people to lead productive lives and to take care of themselves, their families, and their communities, which are all issues of occupational justice (Whiteford & Townsend, 2011).

Inequalities in resource distribution and the problem of poverty

Poverty is a problem throughout the world. In addition, the gap between the rich and the poor is increasing dramatically, affecting the vulnerability of not only poor people but those in the middle class as well (Associated Press, 2008; Primorac, 2011; Rogers & Kamal, 2005). By the year 2005, the 500 world's richest people were earning more than the 416,000,000 poorest people (Rogers & Kamal, 2005). At the same time, "45% of the world's population" lived on US$2.00 or less per day (p. 1). According to the International Monetary Fund (IMF) such income disparities are a concern, not only because extreme inequalities are damaging to the sustainability of any country's economic growth (Primorac, 2011), but also because they unfairly increase the vulnerability of sections of society to dangers arising from the compromised carrying capacity of the earth.

As the ship was sinking in the 1997 movie "*Titanic*", the poor people in the third class were barricaded below decks (in fact, until 1.15 am, [Lord, 1958]) without being given any chance at all to fight for survival while those in the first class boarded life-boats. As Walter Lord remarked in his *A night to remember* (1958, p. 86), "No-one seemed to care about Third Class." It was as if the lives of those in the third class were worthless and needed to be sacrificed for the survival of the worthy wealthy in the first class (ironically, the British Board of Inquiry found that there had been no discrimination). Class distinction was accepted as a fact of life. This is a good metaphor to illustrate the statement by the UNEP (n.d.) that:

> There is a large and widening vulnerability gap between well-off people, with better all-round coping capacity, who are becoming gradually less vulnerable, and the poor who grow increasingly so. It is vital to the sustainable development effort that this gap is addressed, as well as vulnerability itself. (p. 310)

Poor people tend to have fewer resources than the rich at their disposal, and therefore have less coping ability when disasters strike. That is why depletion of resources and eco-damage tends to affect the poor and indigenous communities the most. People in these communities rely more on natural resources and processes and therefore bear the blunt of human-driven climate change. Like the Titanic, as the *SS Earth* sinks as a consequence of the destruction of its eco-support systems, the poor are more likely to die off well before the wealthy. This is certainly a moral and ethical issue to ponder before the Board of Inquiry's post mortem.

Occupational therapists, occupational scientists, and future occupational needs

From the ensuing discussion, some of the pressing issues of concern in current times include: a rapidly growing population; environmental degradation due to unsustainable resource use and environmental abuse; poverty; and increasing income inequalities. If occupational therapists and occupational scientists are to realize the vision of being leaders in society by being science driven, evidence-based, and meeting society's occupational needs, they need to do their part by assuming their proper leadership role in designing occupation-based strategies to contribute towards the solution of the above outlined problems. We have argued in this book that one way of meeting society's occupational needs is by responding to the problem of meaninglessness that Frankl (1992) saw as the most significant challenge of our time. As discussed in earlier chapters, one of the ways in which people derive meaning in life, according to Frankl, is by doing things that increase their connection to a cause that is bigger than them and make them feel that they are contributing to this cause. We put forth the argument in this chapter that there is no bigger cause for someone who wants to make his/her life meaningful than to do one's part in contributing to the restoration of the earth's eco-support systems to ensure survival of future generations. Occupational therapists and scientists can work with people to help them find ways to be personally and collectively accountable to this end by making daily occupational choices in such a way as to ensure that they fulfill their individual obligations in bequeathing a beautiful, life-supporting earth to posterity. To do this, occupational therapists and scientists have to become part of interdisciplinary teams of scientists working to find solutions to these threatening problems.

However, before we can assume our roles in these teams as occupational therapists and scientists, we have to clarify precisely what our contribution to the solution of these problems should be. Detailed examples of such a discussion can be found in Ikiugu (2008). In the present book, we propose that we can make such a contribution in at least two ways: 1) working directly with individuals and small groups within the community; and 2) doing research to inform our understanding of how individual occupational choices and performance patterns affect not only the health of individuals but also how they affect the health of the eco-system and therefore the earth's carrying capacity for human beings.

Working with individuals and groups in the community

In considering how occupational therapists and scientists can work with individuals and groups in communities to address the major issues of our time as discussed above, we first look at: 1) the relationship between occupation and the outlined issues; and 2) how occupation-based approach to solving these issues would help people achieve increased meaning in their lives. First, we would like to emphasize that the issues in question may be viewed as occupational in nature. Taking the environment as an example, the National Academy of Sciences [NAS] (1997) stated the following:

> Environmental policies are influenced by economic, social, and political forces. To ensure that the execution of these policies protects human health and ecosystems effectively, scientific and technical information needs to be an integral consideration from the earliest stages of policymaking. (p. 5 of 15)

It can be said that other major social issues, such as income inequalities, poverty, and governance, are similarly affected by economic, social, and political forces. But if we look at the definition of occupation, it is clear that economic, social, and political forces are essentially occupational in nature. For example, Crepeau, Cohn, and Schell (2003, p. 1030) define occupation as: "daily activities that reflect cultural values, provide structure to living, and meaning to individuals; these activities meet human needs for self-care, enjoyment, and participation in society". Pollard and Sakellariou (2012) further state:

> Every day people orchestrate and perform numerous occupations. Some of them are responses to biological needs, such as eating or sleeping; some are socially required or expected (working, paying bills); some maintain the benefits of a social network and others may simply be fun whether alone or shared with others. (p. 9)

In both these statements, occupation pertains to self-care and productivity including earning a living so that one is able to meet biological needs and physically survive; self-enjoyment or what many may refer to as participation in leisure; and functioning as a social being, which includes working with others to contribute towards meeting common societal needs, which includes political participation or what Kronenberg and Pollard (2005) refer to as political activities of daily living (pADLs).

All the activities delineated above are what underlie economic, social, and political forces. For example, earning a living so that one can sustain oneself physiologically and afford participation in enjoyable leisure activities is an economic endeavor. Addressing issues of collective concern to society or simply socializing by sharing meals constitute social participation, which is defined by the NAS as a social force. Working with others through activities such as participation in town hall meetings, community organizations, or neighbourhood events can influence social policy. Engagement in developing resources such as horticulture projects on allotments, writing groups, local history groups, sports leagues, festivals and concerts are ways of enhancing aspects of community life and building social capital, as well as a means of sharing community life and having fun. All these are the basis for political activities of daily living (pADLs) (Kronenberg & Pollard, 2005; Pollard, Kronenberg, & Sakellariou, 2008).

These pADLs, whether directly 'political', directly 'environmental', or not, have the effect of providing opportunities for people in communities to assess, negotiate, and voice their perceptions regarding local development needs (See Max-Neef, 1991, 2010) which underlie what the NAS calls a political force. Sports leagues need to have safe access to clean playing fields and pollution free air. Allotments have to be managed carefully alongside other allotment users and need to be regularly maintained. Writing and local history groups discuss changes in the community, including changes in the environment and social conditions. Festivals and concerts need space, such as the local park, and have an environmental impact. Thus, all the major issues of our time originate from the human performance of work, self-care, and/or leisure occupations. They can be addressed by people at the grassroots understanding the linkages between their activities and their experiences of these issues, and subsequently taking the opportunity to make informed changes in their occupational behaviors, and consequently ameliorating the issues.

Secondly, as mentioned earlier, by working with people to help them resolve the issues of concern through their occupational choices and performance, occupational therapists and scientists would be helping them contribute to a cause that is bigger than them. People would be individually exercising their agency to contribute to survival and quality of life for posterity which is a great, self-transcendent cause. By exercising their agency in that manner, they would be meeting one of the criteria for meaningful life as defined by Frankl (1992) and as affirmed by occupational therapy leaders such as Yerxa (1967) in her statement that:

> The particular reality of the occupational therapy clinic involves not only the client's disability but his opportunity to make the kinds of choices by which he can discover, for himself, the meaning of his own existence and realize his potentials in accordance with that meaning. Our clinics are one of the few environments within institutions in which the client can make such choices. (p. 137)

Of course what we are proposing in this book is different from Yerxa's conceptualization. For one, we are proposing working with clients and doing research in communities, rather than in institutions. Secondly, we conceptualize the future client as not necessarily having a disability but needing to find a sense of meaning in his/her life. Further, as proposed by the AOTA (2014), the clients will be not only individuals but also communities. Now, having demonstrated that the issues of decreasing carrying capacity of the earth, income inequalities, and poverty are the result of economic, social, and political forces, which are driven by human occupational performance, we now examine what occupational therapists can do to help address them. The NAS (1997) proposed a number of measures to address environmental problems which we think can be adopted by occupational therapists/scientists to address all the delineated issues.

Working with individuals and communities at the grassroots to facilitate action

According to the NAS,

> [the] public participation in risk assessment, risk management, and the projected cost of cleanup can be critical in developing and gaining public acceptance of environmental initiatives. (1997, p. 9)

As an illustration of this public involvement, Anderson (2008) provides a report of a workshop of "disasters roundtable" that was organized by the National Academies. In the round table, various experts began by providing information about the effect of disasters to communities, including the effect of such disasters on the GDP, which can be devastating in poorer countries. During the discussion, roundtable participants examined their own experiences in order to gain insight into the impact of such disasters on them, and then discussed measures that can be taken to address the risks. A similar approach has been used successfully by the Green Belt movement (Maathai, 2010). Explaining how she conducts seminars to encourage women at the grass-roots to get involved in planting trees and restoring the eco-system, Maathai wrote:

> At each seminar, each group enumerates its problems. It is then challenged to explore where those problems came from and how to develop a set of actions it can take to solve them both immediately and in the long term – at individual, household, and community levels, and on a small or larger scale. (p. 28)

Occupational therapists and occupational scientists can use a similar approach to this form of community development. For example, they can work with others to organize seminars with people in the rural communities, focusing on drawing from participants' experiences to promote an understanding of how individual occupational performance relates to the issues of concern. In these seminars, they can challenge participants to explore the problems facing them, such as wetland destruction. Participants can examine how this destruction of wetlands for example affects water aquifers leading to decreased fresh water supply, and how degradation of wetlands also destroys the natural barriers against soil erosion, leading to low agricultural output. They can reflect on how the decreased agricultural output affects them individually economically. Seminar participants can then reflect on how their own occupational choices and performance patterns, for instance draining the wetlands in order to provide building space, or farming along the river-banks, contribute to the problem of wetland destruction. Finally, they can discuss strategies for changing their occupational behaviors individually in order to collectively solve the problem of wetland destruction in their community and thus reverse the land's compromised carrying capacity.

An addition that we would make to Maathai's approach would be to help seminar participants commit to action designed to change occupational behavior by taking them through the process of personal mission establishment as discussed in chapter 6. Such mission statements would help them place their planned changes in occupational lifestyles in the larger context of contributing to a cause that is bigger than them. Concrete actions that people may be encouraged to take would include developing community actions such as art or theatre events, taking pictures, and developing web based blogs. Such contextualization would help seminar participants enhance their sense of meaning in life. A similar approach can be used to address all the problems discussed in this chapter that we see as threatening the very human survival.

Integrating indigenous wisdom

When working with people to develop occupation-based solutions, occupational therapists and scientists need to understand how communities traditionally handled such critical issues. This information would be a way of introducing discussion of viable community-based actions. Taking the issue of environmental protection and restoration as an example, traditionally, indigenous communities had guidelines for environmental conservation. Hayashi (2002) discussed the Japanese approach to environmental conservation as rooted in their traditional view of nature. He suggested that the Asian (and particularly the Japanese) attitude towards the environment was distinctly different from that held by people in the West. The Western attitude towards the environment originated from the Judeo-Christian world view, which took shape in the hostile environment of the desert. Under those circumstances, the environment was seen as a threat and people needed to control it in order to survive. Thus, they conceptualized the resources in the environment as having been given to them by God to harness and control for the benefit of meeting their survival needs. Dominance over the environment became a value in the Western worldview. This pursuit for dominance over the environment may be seen as having largely contributed to its destruction. Many cultures in different parts of the world have collapsed because they over-cultivated land, disrupted their environments, or failed to adapt to natural changes in the ecology (Fernandez-Armesto, 2000). These problems were often in the past confined to local cultures and civilizations, but today we live in an interconnected and global society.

The Japanese on the other hand, according to Hayashi, formulated their world view in a less harsh environment characterized by mountains and forests. Consequently, they saw the environment (actually according to Hayashi, there is no proper Japanese word for the environment since Japanese people do not see themselves as being separate from nature) as both powerful and nurturing. This view was incorporated into their traditional spiritual system of *Shinto* in which *Kami* (the gods) were perceived to reside in nature. Mountains were particularly important for the Japanese because that was where the *Kami* lived and to where the souls of the dead ascended. Therefore, the Japanese had an awe of nature and sought to live in harmony with it rather than to dominate it.

Hayashi points out that in the modern Westernized Japan, that harmonious relationship with nature has been lost, and as Aoyagi-Usui, Vinken, and Kuribayashi (2003) point out, many philosophers have strongly advocated the need for Japanese people to go back to establishing personal relationships with nature, listening to its voice, and living with it rather than fighting against it. The other basis of the world view regarding the human relationship with nature that guides Japanese life even today comes from the fact that Japan is not a resource-rich country. Therefore, people have always understood the need not to be wasteful so as to ensure survival. This attitude is what resulted in the Japanese notion of *Mottainai* (Maathai, 2010; Mottainai Campaign, 2012). *Mottainai* is a lifestyle for the Japanese people in which they strive to respect the environment by using the bounty it provides judiciously. This is achieved by reducing waste, re-using resources, and recycling. Those who subscribe to this lifestyle seek to recognize that we are merely borrowing this earth from future generations and therefore have an obligation to pass on its beauty to them.

In Africa, views of nature that were very similar to those of the Japanese abounded. In many African communities, the gods and goddesses, and a host of spirits, including those of the ancestors, were thought to inhabit nature (Ampadu, n.d.; Eneji et al., 2012; Kanu, n.d.). In Nigeria for example,

> ... the traditional belief system holds the ascription of supernatural powers to objects called gods and goddesses. The major tenet of African traditional religion and belief system lies in the belief that the abode of the gods and goddesses is located in the community, they may decide to have their abodes on rock, streams, pond, trees, land or anywhere else they may decide to live. (Eneji et al., 2012, p. 35)

Similarly, among the Kikuyu (and also the Meru) people of Kenya, when people cleared the land in order to cultivate crops, custom dictated that they practice some form of agroforestry by preserving the larger, straighter trees. Each tree that was left standing was called in Kikuyu, *murema-kiriti*, or "one that resists the cutting of the forest." These trees were considered to be the habitats of the spirits of all the trees that had been cut down. In turn, the standing trees couldn't be felled unless the spirits were transferred to another tree (Maathai, 2010, p. 78).

Through this spiritual worldview, many African communities were required by custom, through various taboos, to conserve the environment. For instance, in the Meru community of Kenya, people were not allowed to encroach on the forests, wetlands, or lakes, because this is where the spirits were believed to live and therefore it was believed that invading such land would be an invasion of the homes of gods and spirits leading to very negative consequences for human beings. In the United States, the Native Americans saw the environment as sacred, and sought to treat it with respect. Thus, their culture included:

> ...numerous ceremonies and rituals with their way of life and showed respect for everything they killed for sustenance. Animals had to be treated properly because they could represent spirits, as well as plants which could give evidence of the supernatural and the land which could reveal God. (Sherrer, n.d., pp. 16-17)

These examples indicate that many indigenous communities had their own solutions to the prevailing global issues, including preservation of the eco-system, which were supported by their cultural and religious worldviews. In many countries, despite increasing cultural diversity, occupational therapists and occupational scientists often represent a narrow social group with cultural experiences that differ from those of many of their clients (Alers, 2010; Beagan, 2007; Danner, Royeen, Martin, Walsh, Royeen, 2011; Shordike, O'Brien, & Marshall, 2011; Simo, 2011). When working with people who may have different cultural backgrounds, occupational therapists and occupational scientists need to discuss and understand these peoples' worldviews, so that they can use effective traditional practices as a point of departure in negotiating with them in the assessment of risk, and formulation of occupational lifestyle interventions to address the issues (Alers, 2010; Barros, Lopes, Galheigo & Galvani 2011; Shordike, O'Brien, & Marshall, 2011).

For example, when working with people of Japanese origin, it may be helpful to help them affirm their lifestyles based on constructs such as *Mottainai* by pointing out to them that such practices benefit them as well as future generations. *Mottainai* may be articulated to Japanese seminar participants as a form of occupational performance in which waste is minimized. For instance, it is customary for Japanese people to exchange gifts when they visit each other (occupational category of social participation). Such gifts are traditionally wrapped in very colorful cloth. The gift recipient uses the same cloth to wrap up a gift to give in return as a token of the friendly relationship. Such practice precludes the wasteful practice of using wrapping paper in the social occupational form of gift exchange.

When working with Africans, it may be useful to discuss how the view of nature as being inhabited by spirits might have originated from a perceived need to conserve natural resources for posterity. The occupational therapist/scientist in this case would need to remember that some African traditions may be based in pantheism and animism but many Africans have been converted to Christian denominations. However, when people need to seek help for issues such as recovery from trauma or mental health problems, or even environment-related problems such as when there is an extended draught, many may turn to traditional healers or religious leaders before resorting to Western scientific approaches (Alers, 2010; Lesunyane, 2010). Working with people in these circumstances to help them see the logical connection between their actions and the issues of concern can be very sensitive. An example of such sensitivity has been noted by therapists working with clients who have HIV/AIDS. In these cases, it has been found that some spiritual counselors may have a rigid and conservative approach which can reinforce the effects of social stigma – yet the client feels a need for spiritual guidance (Van de Reyden & Jourbert, 2005). The point is that traditional approaches need to be taken into consideration if the issues of concern, including environmental issues, have to be addressed effectively.

Church leaders and perhaps other traditional healers may recognize community needs and can play a large role in facilitating community-based, and occupation-based interventions by acting as what Meyer (2010, p. 330) calls a "point of entry". In the process of occupational therapists/scientists developing liaison with clients, it would be critical to respect the value of traditional practices that indigenous people have used for ages to preserve natural resources. It is important to indicate a preparedness to work in ways that respect traditions from the beginning. For example, many African traditions include exchange of gifts in the social discourse in a manner similar to the Japanese culture. Among the Kikuyu and the Meru people of Kenya, when you visited somebody, you brought a gift with you (traditionally carried in the kind of sisal basket mentioned earlier). The host would then put a little gift in the basket and return it to the visitor. Thus, there was no wasteful use of wrapping paper in this social occupational task of gift exchange.

Beginning at the point of entry, bringing along a suitable gift in a traditional sisal basket may enable an occupational therapist or occupational scientist working with people in the Kikuyu and Meru communities to begin a discussion about the plausibility of cultivating small sisal gardens to provide raw materials for use in making baskets and other items. This activity could become the basis of a small social enterprise producing items not only for leisure but also for sale, which might be helpful to poor people in the rural communities of the country (Kiragu, 2011). Thus, people would have an enjoyable leisure occupation that doubles as an ethical source of income. Producing a means of carrying things that does not involve production of pollution could help to reduce the use of plastic bags which are a major element of waste in Kenya. Furthermore, by planting raw materials such as sisal, people would be restoring the carbon sinks and thus helping reduce accumulation of greenhouse gasses in the atmosphere.

In most areas of the world, public engagement with the environmental issues which result from human occupations is quite limited. While people often avow a concern about climate change, they may not follow this up with actions, for example by changing their travel habits or patterns of consumption. Where people may change their behaviours, such as reducing their petrol consumption or recycling their waste, the extent to which they are able to do this is limited by a complex array of factors such as local infrastructures, lack of knowledge and distrust of information, and lack of sufficient income. Thus, environmental measures require policy as well as behavioral change (Semenza et al. 2008; Whitmarsh, Seyfang & O' Neill, 2011). Numerous studies indicate that the effects of climate change and environmental degradation have a greater health and quality of life impact on those with lower incomes (Frumkin, Hess, Luber, Malilay, & McGeehin, 2008; Thomas, Dorling, & Davey Smith, 2010). This issue has an occupational dimension both in terms of the causes of the problem and its consequences. One effective way of developing a coherent approach to addressing environmental needs is to analyze occupations and their impact on global issues, and how such occupations may be used to mitigate the issues.

A significant aspect of present environmentally unsustainable occupational behaviors results from current policy which tends to present responsible consumption as a matter of individual choice (Semenza et al. 2008; Whitmarsh, Seyfang & O' Neill, 2011), while the public health impact of an optional buy-in to environmental concerns produces disparities in life expectancy and quality of life (Frumkin, Hess, Luber, Malilay, & McGeehin, 2008; Thomas, Dorling, & Davey Smith, 2010) thus reducing choice. For many people, the problem is seen as too big to do anything about, and by the time it happens their life will be over anyway. Furthermore, they are concerned about what others will think of them if they change their behavior (Semenza et al. 2008; Seyfang & O' Neill, 2011; Whitmarsh, Seyfang & O' Neill, 2011). If people are to be persuaded to see the logic of increasing chances of survival by changing consumption patterns, conserving natural resources and reducing abuse to the eco-system, there is a need to better understand the belief systems that motivate people's occupational behavior. The development of an applied occupational perspective may provide tools which can assist individuals and communities to make the needed behavior changes. This is the intent of the reflection and information dissemination part of the intervention guided using Ikiugu's Modified Instrumentalism in Occupational Therapy (MIOT) model (Ikiugu, 2011; 2008; Ikiugu & McCollister, 2011) discussed in chapter 6. By applying the *Mottainai* construct widely as a guide to daily occupational performance, human beings could truly transform the planet in very positive ways.

Population management

Toward the end of the last century there was some ambivalence within the occupational therapy profession with regard to recognition of sexual behavior as a legitimate area of practice (Couldrick 1998, 1999). The study of sexual expression and sexuality as aspects of human occupation was not included in the professional education of therapists, and therefore they lacked the necessary skills to formulate interventions to address these issues. Therapists began to call for changes to ensure that clients' needs in this important occupation area were met (Jackson, 1995; Couldrick 1999). More recently, the AOTA (2014) included "sexual activity" in the category of Activities of Daily Living which constitute, "activities that result in sexual satisfaction and/or meet relational or reproductive needs" (s.19). By accepting sexual activity as being within the purview of occupational therapy, occupational therapists and scientists have also to be interested in issues of population management since sexual activity is intimately related to population growth.

Studies have revealed a need for greater involvement of adolescent males and young men in programmes for preventing precocious pregnancy, in place of current measures concentrating on women and girls (Lohan, Cruise, O'Halloran, Alderdice, & Hyde, 2010; Sipsma, Brooks Biello, Cole-Lewis, & Kerhsaw, 2010). The consequences of early fatherhood, including that of precocious parenting, include the tendency for the behavior to be replicated in subsequent generations. These practices in turn have an impact on the quality of life for each generation, since early parenthood often leads to poverty which then becomes a vicious cycle of poverty and poor quality of life that becomes ingrained within the individual's lineage. As Moav (2004) argued, there is a relationship between high fertility rates and the persistence of poverty. He postulated that whereas in wealthy countries there had been a developing trend towards reduced birth-rates with subsequent increased investment in education as life expectancy had increased, poorer countries tended to have traditions of having more children. He presented this as an economic phenomenon of quality versus quantity, with the effect that having more children was related to less capital to invest in each child, leading to replication of poverty. Socioeconomic disadvantage reduces the family capital and can contribute to problems for each child in terms of his life course development. Children from wealthier families are better off than their less wealthy peers with similar educational opportunities. These disparities can be related to the issue of occupational justice.

Letablier, Luci, Math, and Thévenon (2009) agree with Moav (2004) that one way of considering the complex issue of how poverty impacts on children's development may be to consider each child as capital. A child depreciates in capital value with lack of care over time. Therefore, investments have to be made with long term benefits of the positive social benefits of a healthy child in mind. Investment in children corresponds to improvement in the value of the labour supply as each child matures. Schoon and Bynner (2003) point out that the investments needed by poor families in the education of their children is even greater since children from poor families have to perform better than their wealthier peers to attain the same outcomes. Of course one of the ways to ensure maintenance of "child capital" may be by discouraging precocious parenthood which would have an effect of: reducing birth rates; reducing poverty; saving resources that can be invested in the education of the fewer children born to mature parents; and all this would translate into a society that is better equipped to ensure the preservation of the carrying capacity of the planet earth.

Reduction of early sexual activity and attitudes to sexual expression may be one of the domains for occupational therapy intervention. Of course, as Sipsma et al (2010) point out there is a range of factors including drinking, using drugs, dating practices, and opportunities for sexual activity that affect sexual behavior. Never the less, Lohan et al (2010) suggest that there is a need for strategies to engage young people in sex education which goes beyond reproduction. Occupational therapists/scientists can develop strategies for such engagement, which is important considering the implications of sexual activities at a very young age in contributing to unsustainable population growth, not to mention contribution of such activities to other issues such as poverty in society as discussed above.

As Francis-Connolly (1998) found, mothering has lifelong occupational implications. She argued that occupational therapists have tended to concentrate their efforts on interventions focusing on children with disabilities and their families. She argued that they should develop a wider focus for their interventions to include parenting as an occupation. Such broadening of focus is significant given the household expenditure patterns that have been observed in which major budgetary items include housing and utility bills, transportation, food, goods and services. Child care accounts for 20-30% of European household budgets (Letablier, Luci, Math, & Thévenon, 2009), which is an underestimate since figures only include costs associated with children up to age 14. By broadening the scope of their interventions to include parenting, occupational therapists may contribute towards breaking the cycle of precocious parenthood and its consequences including contributing to unsustainable population growth, poverty, and other issues.

Further, occupational therapists/scientists may use Max-Neef's (2010, p. 206) matrix of "needs and satisfiers" as a means of communicating the actual occupational cost of bringing up a child and the effect of each child on the quality of life for all the other children in the family, and for the well-being of the entire society. Once people realistically examine the positive and negative consequences of having children, the impact each child has on the family individually and collectively, and how each additional child impacts on the ability of future children to survive, then they can take the next step of examining how their sexual behavior may expose them to having children for whom they may not have planned. This self-examination can be a basis for change in sexually oriented activities so that people can enjoy sexual satisfaction while ensuring that they have children only when they have adequately planned for them.

Participation in the development of a human-focused economic system

According to Max-Neef (2010), the world's recent economic problems (including extreme income inequalities) are the consequences of application of outdated 19th century economic theories to a 21st century global economy. For example, unlike the assertion by capitalists that the demand and supply dynamics serve human interests overall through creation of wealth, the reality is that the economy does not always supply what is necessary for the well-being of human beings.

This discrepancy, according to Max-Neef, is the product of an economic system in which human-beings serve the economy rather than the other way round. Creating well-being for humanity is no longer the ultimate objective of the economic system. Rather, the system calls for humans to serve it so that it can grow for the sake of its own growth. These issues have a direct influence on health. For example, Morel and Mossialos (2010) have pointed to the need to develop new antibiotics. The rate at which infectious diseases are evolving is outpacing the development of antibiotics. However, because we function in an economic system that requires people to work to prompt it up for its own sake rather than the system producing goods that people need, pharmaceutical companies are not supporting research to generate new antibiotics because the limited evidence of their effectiveness means that new medicines are used only as a last resort. Therefore, new drugs are not used in sufficient quantities to defray research costs or to generate profits. Since they are not currently profitable, many pharmaceutical companies do not see the need to invest in them.

In addition, Sutherland et al. (2008, p. 821) identified a range of "future novel threats" to the UK's biodiversity, some of which came from technological innovations in which genetic characteristics may be transferred between organisms leading to new pathogens in the process of commercial research. Further, climate change is becoming increasingly recognized as a chief threat to global health (WHO 2003). Sutherland et al. (2008) made the point that a strategy needed to be developed to explain the need for biodiversity and action on climate change in financial terms, so as to bring major financial interests on board, so as to have any chance of success in confronting these issues. These threats are not currently being addressed because we have an economic system that is not geared towards the well-being of humanity, but rather towards maximizing profits irrespective of where those profits come from, or the extent to which activities necessary to make those profits threaten human survival in the long run.

Max-Neef calls for a new economic model in which people are prioritized over objects and therefore the system serves human beings rather than the other way round. Such a system would require a new economic unit of measurement. He proposed the Genuine Progress Indicator (GPI) as the new unit that would measure overall human well-being that is produced by the economic activities. The GPI would replace the Gross Domestic Product (GDP) which typically does not distinguish between economic activities that are "good" from those that are "bad" for human well-being. We propose that occupational therapists and occupational scientists can significantly contribute to the development of an occupation-based development of such a unit of economic activity measurement. They can help develop new instruments to measure and track Genuine Progress by assessing the extent to which participation in economic activities enhances: *connection* to the environment and to other people; *creative* service and contribution to the well-being of posterity; and increase in the level of happiness and overall sense of well-being in society.

Conducting research

The NAS (1997) emphasized the view that policy-making to address the environmental problems must be based on a good scientific and technical understanding of the underlying issues, whether for population management, income inequalities, poverty, or environmental changes. The effects of human occupational activity are generating multiple changes, from the acidification of the oceans to deforestation, to the increased tendency for flash flooding in built environments or increases in fires. The causation of these issues is complex, and as indicated in the discussion above, effective intervention to address the issues involves providing as much information as possible to people. If people are to assess the risk involved in the issues and make action choices, they need to have reliable information on which to base their decisions. Occupational therapists and scientists must generate the theoretical explanation and evidence connecting occupational performance to the issues in question.

Research questions that need to be answered in order to generate necessary theory and empirical evidence on which people can act include the following: What are the relationships among individual occupational performance, human health, and environmental/ecological health? How do human occupational choices in productivity, self-care, and leisure affect the accumulation of greenhouse gases and degradation of the tropospheric ozone layer, or the build-up of plastic waste in the oceans? What changes in individual occupational choices would lead to a threshold so that momentum is created to decrease ozone depletion significantly?

What are the relationships among individual consumer habits in the process of engaging in productivity, self-care, and leisure, and accumulation of greenhouse gasses in the atmosphere?

Making it So

Where are we going to get the Resources to Expand the Scope of Practice?
One important question that obviously arises is: What is the feasibility of expanding the scope of practice and scholarship for occupational therapists and scientists as discussed in this book? For example, given that the profession has 350,000 members worldwide (www.WFOT.org.au), equivalent to the population of Malta, from where will occupational therapists and scientists get the resources needed for the community-based interventions proposed here? Higgs and Titchen (2001) offered a discussion on the direction of the knowledge-practice interface in occupational therapy which hinted at some of the issues we have addressed in this book. One of their suggestions for education and training was to address the interpersonal as well as the clinical needs, and to focus on the issues that arise from engagements with patients, families and communities in practice. They recognised that the context of practice was fluid and complex, and knowledge and practice in the context had to evolve. Their concern was that occupational therapists were being influenced too much in their development by political and funding decisions rather than by professional values.

However political and funding decisions are often themselves affected by popular demands in the population. Occupational therapists and occupational scientists need to generate more awareness of their potential value to the community in order to ensure that their interventions and services are in demand by the public which subsequently would influence politicians and decision makers in their favor. Kronenberg, Pollard, and Simo Algado (2005), Pollard, Sakellariou, and Kronenberg (2008), Kronenberg, Pollard, and Sakellariou (2011), and Thew, Edwards, Baptiste and Molineux (2011) give examples of a range of occupational therapists' experiences that illustrate the expanding professional scope for occupational therapy, where cases of occupational therapists working with groups using occupation-based interventions are illustrated. These new arenas of practice, in the community, can provide opportunities to advocate for social support of community-based programs and scholarship to address the issues of concern introduced in this chapter (Simo, 2011), through pADLs (Kronenberg & Pollard 2005; Pollard, Kronenberg & Sakellariou, 2008). A potential example of how everyday activities may contribute to scholarship is a call by Husk, Lovell, Cooper, Garside (2013), who are seeking evidence from a broad range of sources in the Cochrane Review supporting the hypothesis that "environmental enhancement and conservation activities" benefit physical and mental health of people. Their intended review is based on the recognition that valuable evidence may be found in projects where a variety of occupational therapists and scientists have been working with people from low incomes groups and with clients with mental health problems.

The second point is that technology makes it possible to begin programs and publicize them quite cheaply and effectively. For example, the seminars suggested earlier can be organized and conducted in a traditional face to face setting, but they can also be conducted at nominal cost through social media such as facebook, blogs, or smartphones. Once people begin participating, forming groups, or developing programs, it might be easier to solicit financial support or support in kind (for example, the provision of spaces to meet, help with administration, supplies of stationery) for further actions, whether more face to face seminars, or support for projects. Thus, there are many creative ways that occupational therapists and occupational scientists can use to get started in necessary programming and scholarship.

Expanding the profession's scope of practice

The proposals made in this book call for occupational therapists and occupational scientists to take a leap and venture beyond the current scope of practice and scholarship, but such a departure may at the same time be seen as consolidating aspects of our underpinning knowledge. Though such a leap may seem disconcerting to many occupational therapists and scientists, an occupation-based approach has to take account of changes in the way that health and social care, and its traditional area of activity, are being conceived. There is a risk that occupational therapy could be relegated to historical irrelevance because it has not been well understood by managers, by other medical professionals, and at times by its sister professions in allied health and nursing professions. It is time to be bold and take a chance.

When Pinel (1962) decided to revolutionize mental health care by using occupations as a means of managing patients instead of chaining them, the then medical establishment was probably rather skeptical. We know for sure that in York, England, Tuke (1964) faced resistance in his attempt to establish a mental health care facility using occupation-based moral treatment principles. His ideas were initially rejected and he was successful only because he persisted. Without the courage of those forefathers and foremothers of the profession, occupational therapy would most probably not even exist today. Occupational therapists and occupational scientists face a continuing challenge to demonstrate the value and prestige of their profession and scientific discipline in society.

Conclusion

In this chapter, we began by pointing out that occupational therapists and scientists are seeking wider societal recognition. This is illustrated by the AOTA vision for occupational therapy to become a science-based and evidence-based profession that meets society's occupational needs. We argued that in order to be recognized, occupational therapy and occupational science need to investigate and develop ways of helping all people construct meaning in their lives through daily occupations. If in the 1960s, Gene Rodenberry, the producer of the long running *Star Trek* series had encountered Mary Reilly (1962), occupational therapy would really have been recognized as the greatest idea of the 21st century. In the *USS Enterprise* medical team, alongside Dr. McCoy, the diverse crew would have included a versatile occupational therapist who facilitated appropriate occupational interventions amongst the ship's contingent during long deep space voyages, and during the later series the crew might have acquired an occupational scientist to offer insights into the problems encountered in the starship's many community based engagements with alien populations on distant planets. In subsequent generations, the future of the galaxy would have been defined in many occupational dimensions, extending the concept of holism into a new universality.

Along with mobile phones, automatic sliding doors and flat screen visual displays that featured as popular, taken for granted innovations in the science fiction of the 1960s, occupation based technologies and assessments could have become a standard component of everyday life in the present. But this can still happen. As Viktor Frankl's work indicates, one of the ways of creating meaningful existence is by helping people connect to and contribute to a reality that is bigger than them. This view is consistent with the occupational therapists' recognition that there is no limit to human potential. We suggested in this book that there is no larger cause for human beings than taking measures to ensure survival of the human species far into the future. We can help people contribute towards that cause by helping them change their occupational lifestyles so that they choose and engage in occupations in such a way as to enhance the human carrying capacity of the earth. Such measures would include occupation-based interventions for environmental and eco-support protection and restoration, occupation-based population management approaches, and participation in political Activities of Daily Living (pADLs). In designing such occupation-based interventions to address the issues of concern, occupational therapists and occupational scientists need to work with individuals and groups in communities. In so doing they will contribute to further breakthroughs and developments in the profession and discipline.

Glossary of Terms

Context: The physical environment or period of time in which a person engages in the process of meaning-making.

Developmental Stage: This term refers to periods of time during which individuals fulfill specific developmental tasks necessary for successful adaptation to changing life circumstances and social participation. Levinson (1978) differentiated between stable and transitional stages: while he saw adolescence as a transitional stage on the way to adult status, the midlife prefaced a stable older adulthood. As Levinson focused exclusively on the midlife rather than development through the lifespan we have not specified this distinction here.

Developmental Task: This term is defined by Havighurst (1982, 1972, 1952) to mean a critical task that arises in one's life at specific times, and whose mastery is satisfying to the individual and facilitates adaptation and transition to the next stage. For example, engagement in school activities is a task of childhood whose mastery may be satisfying to the individual and facilitates successful transition to the adolescence stage. We have conceptualised the human transition through life metaphorically as a journey. As discussed in chapter four, the vehicles employed in that journey include belief supporting institutions such as culture and religion, and intellectual pursuits through activities such as philosophizing or engaging in scientific inquiry.

Developmental stages can be compared to train stations, harbor docks, bus stages, or airports, where the vehicle for transportation stops for boarding or for passengers to refresh themselves. In these stations, the sources of meaning (refreshments if we continue with our metaphor) include establishment of *emotionally intense relationships*, participating in *work and leisure activities*, and *adhering to idea systems*. From these sources, the individual experiences meaning in four dimensions: *sense of self-worth, experience of having a purpose in life, sense of control in one's life circumstances*, and a feeling that one has the ability to express *personal values* effectively and satisfactorily in life. At each station or stage in life, individuals engage in developmental tasks which are revealed from these three sources and four dimensions of meaning.

Dimensions of meaning: Avenues through which people experience a sense of meaning in their lives, including feelings of efficacy, belonging, and having a sense of purpose in life.

Desirable Consequences: Results of one's actions that meet his/her need to construct, destroy, rejuvenate, and inhabit the world, and therefore survive.

Every-Day Occupations: Things people do every day to occupy their time including activities related to taking care of themselves, enjoying themselves, earning a living, and contributing to the welfare of others and of their communities/society [American Occupation Therapy Association (AOTA), 2014; Canadian Occupational Therapists Association (CAOT, 2002)].

Existential Vacuum: A sense of emptiness in one's existence due to loss of connection to the natural environment; grounding in traditions, religion, or philosophy; and lack of connection to something experienced as bigger than oneself.

Experiential Definition of Meaning: Meaning is a manifestation of actions that result in consequences perceived as desirable in one's life.

God-Centered Meaning: Perception of meaning as resulting from being in a relationship with a higher being who is infinite, perfect, and whom many people refer to as God.

Idea Systems: Systems characterized by doctrines, ideologies, or bodies of thought that are propagated to the adherents and provide a unique identity for them. Such systems may be religious, political, social, or cultural.

Leisure: Things people do to enjoy themselves, such as quiet and active recreation (reading a book, painting, engaging in sports, hiking, and others), hobbies (including crafts) or any other activities engaged in purely for recreation. In this definition, it is recognized that sometimes the boundaries between work and leisure may be blurred. For example, a basketball player may enjoy the game and achieve recreation from engaging in it (which qualifies it as leisure) but also earn a living from it. Also, it is recognized that in some cultures, there is no category of activities specifically designated as leisure. The above definition refers to the Western conceptualization of leisure. This is however not to suggest that non-Western cultures lack recreational activities. Communal events, festivities, and other similar activities sustain cultural life through the enjoyment and appreciation of foods, music, telling stories, and other aspects of human relationships, and therefore they are recreational or leisure activities. However they are considered differently because they may contain spiritual significance.

At the same time the process of globalization is spreading the Western concept of leisure into other cultures along with other influences.

Meaning – General Definition: The ability to make sense of reality of one's experience; a sense that one's life is coherent, has order and harmony, and is valuable, and that one is able to make decisions and act upon them and therefore is in control of his or her life.

Meaning as a Creative Endeavor: The notion that meaning emerges from engagement in creative activities.

Meaningful Living: Organization of one's activities to maximize the experience of life as full, valuable, and purposeful.

Soul-Centered Meaning: Experience of meaningfulness as resulting from engagement in activities that facilitate expression of one's eternal soul or spirit.

Objective Meaning: Subsuming external criteria by which a person's life may be objectively judged as meaningful.

Subjective Meaning: The view that meaning is based on each individual's idiosyncratic interpretation of his/her reality.

Meaninglessness: The feeling that one's life is senseless, incoherent, empty, and lacking in value and purpose.

Meaning-making: A process consisting of measures people take to cultivate a sense of meaning and purpose in their lives.

Noogenic Neurosis: Experience of anxiety that results from existential vacuum resulting in meaninglessness as defined above.

Participation: This refers to the process of living life by engaging in the community through performance of occupations that enable one to communicate and relate to other people, take care of him/herself, and generally contribute to the improvement of the lives of other people in the community including family members.

Primary control: The sense that one is in control of the environment across the spectrum of areas of his/her life and over the lifespan, and therefore can influence or determine the direction of his/her life course through specific choices and actions (Heckhausen, Schulz, & Wrosch, 2010).

Quest for Meaning: The process of meaning-making in life is visualized in this book using the metaphor of embarking on a journey, which begins with birth and ends with death. It is the actions that a person takes during this journey that imbue life with meaning. This means that finding meaning is not absolute. One never really arrives at the destination (a place where life meaning is finally realized). Rather, meaning-making is a continuous process that emerges from the continuous process of making choices and acting on those choices.

Transitions: Environmental (as when a person moves from one environmental context to another), temporal (one's transition through time such as the current transition through a temporal period of economic recession), or developmental (one's negotiation of developmental stages from childhood through death).

Vehicles used in the Quest for Meaning: Cultural artifacts, learning, social relationships, etc. are not meaningful unto themselves. It is what they symbolize to the individual that makes an individual's life meaningful. Therefore, they are simply means to an end. A person uses these avenues to create meaning in his/her life, hence, they are merely vessels or vehicles that one uses in his/her quest for meaning in life.

Work – As used in this book, work refers to things that people do to earn a living, to be productive, or to contribute to the well-being of other people around them, their communities, and their society. By this definition, work includes among other things working for wages, volunteering, doing home management, taking care of children, taking care of the elderly, and other related activities. However, while attempting to define this construct, it should be recognized that not all work is productive and its context can often be exploitive. For example, the second author previously worked in the betting industry as a cashier, taking bets on sports events. Betting can be seen as a leisure occupation for people who may be entertained through gambling as an occupation. However many of the customers clearly had problems with their betting behavior, from which the company made profits. This was exploitation, and neither socially productive nor a contribution to the well-being of those people. Similarly, many jobs in the current economy lack opportunities for progression, are low paying, unsafe, insecure, contribute to ill-health and place pressures on individuals' family life and relationships (Grimshaw, Carroll, & Rubery 2008).

References

Abberley, P. (1995). 'Disabling Ideology in Health and Welfare -the case of occupational Therapy'. *Disability & Society.* 10(2), 221-232

Abbott, D. (2012). Nudge, nudge, wink, wink: love, sex and gay men with intellectual disabilities – a helping hand or a human right? *Journal of Intellectual Disability Research.* DOI: 10.1111/j.1365-2788.2012.01642.x

Abrahams, T. (2008). Occupation, identity and choice: A dynamic interaction. *Journal of Occupational Science, 15*(3), 186-189

Adamczyk, A. L. (2005). Frankl, Bettelheim and the camps. *Journal of Genocide Research,* 7(1), 67-84.

Adams, C. (Ed). (1987). *Across seven seas and thirteen rivers.* London: Tower Hamlets Arts Project.

Adams, D. (1979). *The hitchhikers guide to the galaxy.* London: Pan.

Addis, M. E., Hatgis, C., Cardemil, E., Jacob, K., Krasnow, A. D., & Mansfield, A. (2006). Effectiveness of cognitive-behavioral treatment for panic disorder versus treatment as usual in a managed care setting: 2-year follow-up. *Journal of Consulting and Clinical Psychology, 74*(2), 377-385.

Aguilar, A., Boerema, C., & Harrison, J. (in press). Meaning attributed by older adults to computer use. *Journal of Occupational Science.*

Akter, K. (1998). *Oceans apart.* Manchester: Gatehouse.

Alers, V. (2010). Working with trauma survivors – from victim to trauma survivor to thriver. In V. Alers & R Crouch (eds.) *Occupational Therapy: an African perspective.* (pp 268-284). Johannesburg: Sarah Shorten.

Allan, G. (1989). *Friendship: developing a sociological perspective.* New York: Harvester Wheatsheaf.

Alspach, R. K. (1943). Some sources of Yeats's *The wanderings of Oisin. PMLA, 58*(3), 849-866.

American Occupational Therapy Association. (2006). *AOTA's centennial vision.* Found at http://www.aota.org/nonmembers/area16/index.asp.

American Occupational Therapy Association. (2014). Occupational therapy practice framework: Domain & process (3rd ed.). *American Journal of Occupational Therapy,* 68(Supplement 1), S1-S51.

Ampadu, C. (n.d.). *Correlation between African traditional religions and the problems of African societies today.* Accra, University of Ghana. Found at http://www.wciu.edu/docs/general/ampadu_article.pdf.

Anderson, W. A. (Ed.). (2008). *Disaster risk management in an age of climate change: A summary of the April 3, 2008 workshop of the disasters roundtable.* National Academy of Sciences. Found at http://www.nap.edu/catalog.php?record_id=12575.

Aoyagi-Usui, M., Vinken, H., & Kuribayashi, A. (2003). Pro-environmental attitudes and behaviors: An international comparison. *Human Ecology Review, 10*(1), 23-31.

Arbesman, M., & Mosley, L. J. (2012). Systematic review of occupation-and activity-based health management and maintenance interventions for community-dwelling older adults. *American Journal of Occupational Therapy, 66*, 277-283.

Ariew, A. (n.d.). *Patonic and Aristotelian roots of teleological arguments in cosmology and biology*. Retrieved on January 3, 2013 from web.missouri.edu/-ariewa/Teleology/.pdf.

Arnett, J. J. (2000). Emerging adulthood: A theory of development from the late teens through the twenties. *American Psychologist, 55*, 469-480.

Arnett, J. J., & Tanner, J. L. (Eds.). (2006). *Emerging adults in America: Coming of age in the 21st century*. Washington, DC: American Psychological Association.

Associated Press. (2008, October 21). *Study: Gap growing between rich and poor* [Electronic Version]. Retrieved August 8, 2012, from http:www.msnbc.msn.com/id/27295405/ns/business-world_business/t/study-gap-growing-...

Baker, J. (1985) *A mis-spent youth.* Hackney, Centerprise

Barber, M. (1999). *A life behind bars.* Brighton, UK: QueenSpark.

Barnes, R. (1976). *Coronation cups and jam jars.* Hackney, UK: Centerprise.

Barr, J. (1992). *The garden of Eden and the hope of immortality.* London: SCM.

Barros, D.D. Lopes, R.E., Galheigo, S.M. & Galvani, D. (2011) Research, community-based projects, and teaching as a sharing construction: the Metuia Project in Brazil. In F. Kronenberg, N. Pollard, & D. Sakellariou (Eds.), *Occupational therapies without borders* (pp. 332-337). London: Churchill Livingstone/Elsevier.

Bates, D. G., & Plog, F. (1990). *Cultural anthropology.* New York: McGraw Hill.

Bayley, J. (1967). Introduction to *Great short works of Tolstoy.* New York: Harper & Row.

Beagan, B. L. (2007). Experiences of social class: learning from occupational therapy students. *Canadian Journal of Occupational Therapy, 74*, 125-33.

Beagan, B. L., & Chacala, A. (2012). Culture and diversity among occupational therapists in Ireland: when the therapist is the 'diverse' one. *British Journal of Occupational Therapy, 75*(3), 144-151.

Beavis, D. (1980). *What price happiness? My life from coal hewer to shop steward.* Whitley Bay, UK: Strong Words.

Beckman, M. (1992). *The 43 group, the untold story of their fight against fascism.* Hackney, UK: Centerprise.

Belliotti, R. A. (2001). *What is the meaning of life?* Amsterdam-Atlanta, GA: Rodopi.

Berger, P.L. (1973). *The social reality of religion.* Harmondsworth: Penguin.

Berne, E. (1964). *The games people play.* Harmondsworth: Penguin.

Bettelheim, B. (1970). *The informed heart.* London: Paladin.

Black, M. (2011). From kites to kitchens: Collaborative community-based occupational therapy with refugee survivors of torture. In F. Kronenberg, N. Pollard, & D. Sakellariou (Eds.), *Occupational therapies without borders* (Vol 2, pp. 217-225). New York: Churchill Livingstone/Elsevier.

Blakely, J., & Ribiero, V. (2008). Are nurses prepared for retirement. *Journal of Nursing Management. 16*(6), 744-752.

Block, P., Shuttleworth, R., Pratt, J., Block, H., & Rammler, L. (2012). Disability,

Sexuality and Intimacy. In N. Pollard & D. Sakellariou Eds, *Politics of Occupation-Centred Practice* (pp.162-177). Oxford: Wiley.

Bockoven, J.S. (1971). Occupational therapy -A historical perspective: Legacy of moral treatment 1800s to 1910. *American Journal of Occupational Therapy, 25*, 233-225.

Bourdieu, P. (1986). "Forms of Capital", in John G. Richardson (ed.), *Handbook of Theory and Research for the Sociology of Education* (pp241-258). New York: Greenwood.

Bowlby, J. (1980). *Attachment and loss: Vol. 3. Loss: Depression and sadness*. New York: Basic Books.

Bowlby, J. (1982). *Attachment and loss, vol. 1: Attachment* (2nd ed.). New York: Basic Books.

Briar, C. (2006). 'Babies and Bosses'. *Journal of Feminist Family Therapy, 17*(3), 47-65.

Brighton Ourstory Project. (1992). *Daring hearts. Lesbian and Gay lives of 50s and 60s Brighton*. Brighton, UK: QueenSpark.

Bristol Broadsides. (1987). *Bristol lives*. Bristol, UK: author.

Bristol Broadsides. (1988). *More Bristol lives*. Bristol, UK: author.

British Broadcasting Corporation. (2011, August). The competing arguments used to explain the riots [online version]. *BBC News Magazine*. Retrieved January 2nd, 2013, from www.bbc.co.uk/news/magazine-14483149.

Brogan, H. (1990). *The Penguin history of the United States of America*. London: Penguin.

Brown, J., Hanlon, P., Turok, I., Webster, D., Arnott, J., & Macdonald, E. B. (2008). Establishing the potential for using routine data on Incapacity Benefit to assess the local impact of policy initiatives. *Journal of Public Health, 30*(1), 54-59.

Bruni, L. (2006). *Civil happiness: Economics and human flourishing in historical perspective*. New York: Routledge.

Buchan, D. (1997). *The ballad and the folk*. East Linton: Tuckwell Press.

Butcher, H.K., & McGonigal-Kenney, M. (2005). Depression & Dispiritedness in Later Life: A 'gray drizzle of horror' isn't inevitable. *American Journal of Nursing*: 105(12), 52-61

Canadian Association of Occupational Therapists. (2002). *Enabling occupation: An occupational therapy perspective*. Ottawa, ON: CAOT Publications ACE.

Cannadine, D. (1983). The context, performance and meaning of ritual: the British monarchy and the invention of tradition c1820-1977. In E. Hobsbawm, & T. Ranger (Eds.), *The invention of tradition* (pp. 101-164). Cambridge: Cambridge University Press.

Capra, F. (1996). *The web of life: A new scientific understanding of living systems*. New York: Doubleday.

Capra, F. (1999). *The tao of physics: An exploration of the parallels between modern physics and Eastern mysticism*. Boston: Shambhala.

Capstick, S. (1988). *A woman's right to cues*. Castleford, UK: Yorkshire Arts Circus.

Carlson, M., Clark, F., & Young, B. (1998). Practical contributions of occupational science to the art of successful ageing: How to sculpt a meaningful life in older adulthood. *Journal of Occupational Science, 5*(3), 107-118.

Carter, D. (1992). *Just one of a large family*. Brighton, UK: QueenSpark.

Cavanagh, K., Shapiro, D. A., van Den Bergl, S., Swain, S., Barkham, M., & Proudfoot,

J. (2006). The effectiveness of computerized cognitive behavioural therapy in routine care. *British Journal of Clinical Psychology, 45*, 499–514

Cech, D. J., & Martin, S. (2002). *Functional movement development across the lifespan* (2nd ed.). Philadelphia: W. B. Saunders.

Centerprise. (n.d.). (ed) (*Working Lives Volume One: 1905-45.* Hackney, UK: Hackney WEA/Centerprise.

Centerprise. (1984). (ed) *Breaking the silence, writing by Asian women.* Hackney, UK: Centerprise.

Centerprise. (1978). *Working Lives Volume Two: People's autobiography of Hackney 1945-77.* Hackney, UK: Hackney WEA/Centerprise.

Chinen, A. B. (1990). *In the ever after: Fairy tales and the second half of life.* Wilmette, IL: Chiron Publications.

Chiriac, J. (2007). *Psychoanalysis and fairy-tales* (Electronic version]. Retrieved April 20, 2008,from http://www.fredufile.org/psychoanalysis/fairy_tales.html.

Chodorow, N. (1978). *The reproduction of mothering, psychoanalysis and the sociology of gender.* Berkley CA: University of California.

Chodorow, N. (1989). *Feminism and psychoanalytic theory.* New Haven: Yale University Press.

Christiansen, C. (1994). Classification and study in occupation: A review and discussion of taxonomies. *Journal of Occupational Science, 1*(3), 3-20.

Christiansen, C. H. (1999). Defining lives: occupation as identity: *an essay on competence, coherence,and the creation of meaning. American Journal of Occupational Therapy, 53,* 547–558.

Christiansen, C. H. (2000): Identity, personal projects and happiness: Self construction in everyday action, *Journal of Occupational Science*, 7:3, 98-107.

Christie, D., & Viner, R. (2005). ABC of adolescent development. *British Medical Journal, 330*, 301-304.

Cicirelli, V. G. (2010). Attachment relationships in old age. *Journal of Social and Personal Relationships, 27*(2), 191-199.

Clapson, M. (2004). *A social history of Milton Keynes: Middle England/edge city.* London: Frank Cass.

Clark, F., Parham, D., Carlson, M. E., Frank, G., Jackson, J., Peirce, D. et al. (1991). Occupational science: Academic innovation in the service of occupational therapy's future. *American Journal of Occupational Therapy, 45,* 300-310.

Clark, F., Jackson, J., Carlson, M., Chou, C-P., Cherry, B. J., Jordan-Marsh, M., Azen, S. P. (2011). Effectiveness of a lifestyle intervention in promoting the well-being of independently living older people: Results of the well elderly 2 randomized controlled trial. *Journal of Epidemiology and Community Health* [online version], 1-9. DOI: 10.1136/jech.2009.099754.

Clemence, A., Karmaniola, A., & Green, E. G. (2007). Disturbing life events and wellbeing after 80 years of age: A longitudinal comparison of survivors and the deceased over five years. *Aging & Society, 27*, 195-213.

Cohen, H. A. (1989). *Bagels with babushka.* Manchester, UK: Gatehouse.

Cohen, S. J., Barret, R., Irlbacher, S., Kertland, P., Mortch, L., Pinter, L., et al. (1997). Executive summary. In S. J. Cohen (Ed.), *The Mackenzie basin impact study (MBIS) final report*. Ottawa, ON: Environment Canada.

Cole, M. B., & Tufano, R. (2008). *Applied theories in occupational therapy: A practical approach*. Thorofare, NJ: Slack

Congar, Y. (2004). *The meaning of tradition*. Ft. Collins, CO: Ignatius Press.

Connor. M.J., & Walton, J.A. (2011). Demoralization and remoralization: a review of these constructs in the healthcare literature. *Nursing Inquiry* 18: 2–11

Cook, G. A. (1983). *A Hackney memory chest*. Hackney, UK: Centerprise.

Copper, B. (1975). *A song for every season*. Frogmore: Paladin.

Corcoran, M. A. (2004). Work, occupation, and occupational therapy. *American Journal of Occupational Therapy, 58*, 367-368.

Couldrick, L. (1998). Sexual Issues within Occupational Therapy Part 1: Attitudes and Practice. *British Journal of Occupational Therapy*. 61(12), 538-544

Couldrick, L. (1999). Sexual Issues within Occupational Therapy Part 2: Implications for Education and Practice. *British Journal of Occupational Therapy*. 62(1), 26-30

Countryman, E. (1986). *The American Revolution*. Edinburgh: I B Tauris.

Crepeau, E., Cohn, E., & Schell, B. (Eds.). (2003). *Willard and Spackman's occupational therapy*. Philadelphia: Lippincott Williams & Wilkins.

Curley, C. (1993). *The cardigan*. Manchester, UK: Gatehouse.

Daily, G. C., & Ehrlich, P. R. (1992, November). Population, sustainability, and earth's carrying capacity: A framework for estimating population sizes and lifestyles that could be sustained without undermining future generations [Electronic Version]. *BioScience*. Retrieved August 2, 2012, from http://dieoff.org/page112.htm.

Dalley, K. (1998). *A daughter of the state*. Brighton, UK: QueenSpark.

Danner, T.C., Royeen, C., Barney, K., Walsh, S.R., Royeen, M. (2011). The occupation of city walking: crossing the invisible line. In F. Kronenberg, N. Pollard, & D. Sakellariou (Eds.), *Occupational therapies without borders* (pp. 393-398). London: Churchill Livingstone/Elsevier.

Davies, I. (1991). *Writing in prison*. Oxford: Blackwell.

Davis, J. A., & Polatajko, H. J. (2010). Occupational development. In C. H. Christiansen & E. A. Townsend (Eds.), *Introduction to occupation: The art and science of living* (pp. 135-174). Upper Saddle River, NJ: Pearson.

Dawkins, R. (2010, May 7). Did religion have an evolutionary value? *Fora Television, Daily*

Motion. Found at www.dailymotion.com/video/xgjkww_dawkins-did-religion-have-an-evolution. Retrieved June 29, 2013.

Dawkins, R. (2008). *The God delusion*. Chicago, IL: Houghton Mifflin Harcourt Publishing Company.

Dawkins, R. (2006). *The selfish gene*. London: Oxford University Press.

De Certeau, M. (1988). *The practice of everyday life*. (trans, S. Rendall). Berkley, CA: University of California.

De Certeau, M., Giard, L., & Mayol, P. (1998). *The practice of everyday life. Volume 2:*

Living and cooking. (Trans, T. Tomasik). Minneapolis, Minnesota: University of Minnesota.

Degalle, M. (2006). Introduction, Buddhism, conflict and violence. In M. Degalle (ed) *Buddhism, conflict and violence in modern Sri-Lanka.* (p1-21) Abingdon: Routledge.

Depaepe, M. (2007). Philosophy and history of education: Time to bridge the gap? *Educational Philosophy and Theory,* doi:10.1111/j.1469-5812.2007.00236.x.

Detweiler, J., & Peyton, C. (1999). Defining occupations: A chronotypic study of narrative genres in a health discipline's emergence. *Written Communication 16,* 412 – 468.

Dewey.J. (1910). "The Influence of Darwin on Philosophy", in *The Influence of Darwin on Philosophy and Other Essays.* (pp 1-19). New York: Henry Holt and Company.

Donahue, W. (1951) Experiments in the education of older adults. *Adult Education Quarterly, 2(*2), 49-59.

Dwyer, L., Nordenfelt, L., & Ternestedt, B. (2008). Three nursing home residents speak about meaning at the end of life. *Nursing Ethics, 15*(1), 97-109.

Dorling, D. (2011). *Injustice: Why social inequality persists.* Cambridge: Policy Press.

do Rozario, L. (1994). Ritual, meaning and transcendence: The role of occupation in modern life. *Journal of Occupational Science, 1*(3), 46-53.

Dresser, M. (1986). *Black and white on the buses: the 1963 colour bar dispute in Bristol.* Bristol: Bristol Broadsides.

Drucker, P. F. (1993). *Post-capitalist society.* New York: Harper Business.

Duncan, S., Alexander, C. & Edwards, R. (2010) What's the problem with teenage parents. In S.

Edwards, D. R., & Alexander, C. (Eds.). *Teenage parents: What's the problem?* (pp. 1-23). London: The Tufnell Press.

Dunn, R. (1990). *Moulsecoomb Days.* Brighton, UK: QueenSpark.

Du Toit, V. (2009). *Patient volition and action in occupational therapy.* Pretoria: Vona and Marie du Toit Foundation.

Duxbury, L., Lyons, S. & Higgins, C. (2008). Too much to do and not enough time: an examination of work-overload. In K. Korabik, D. S. Leron & D. L. Whitehead (Eds.), *Handbook of work-family integration: research, theory and best practices* (pp 125- 140). London: Academic Press.

Dwyer, L., Nordenfelt, L., & Ternestedt, B. (2008). Three nursing home residents speak about meaning at the end of life. *Nursing ethics, 15*(1), 97-109.

Earl Marshall School. (1993). *Lives of Love and Hope: a Sheffield herstory.* Sheffield,UK: Author.

Edwards, D. L. (1984). *Christian England, volume 3. From the 18th century to the first world war.* London: Collins.

Ehn B., & Lofgren, O. (2010) *The secret world of doing nothing.* Berkley: University of California

Elekes, S. (2011). The role of experiencing meaningfulness related to religious faith in physical wellbeing. *Studia Universitatis Babes-Bolyai, Theological Catholica Latina, LVI* (1), 81-94.

Eneji, C. V., Ntamu, G. U., Ajor, J. O., Ben, C. B., Bassey, J. E., & Williams, J. J. (2012). Ethical basis of African traditional religion and socio-cultural practices in natural resources conservation and management in cross river state, Nigeria. *Journal of Research in Peace, Gender and Development*, 2(2), 34-43.

Erikson, E. H. (1950). *Childhood and society*. New York: Norton.

Erikson, E. H. (1956). The problem of ego identity. *Journal of the American Psychoanalytic Association, 4*, 56-121.

Erikson, E. H. (1963). *Childhood and society* (2nd ed.). New York: Norton.

Erikson, E. H. (1968). *Identity: Youth and crisis*. New York: Norton.

Erikson, E. H. (1975). *Life history and the historical moment*. New York: Norton.

Erikson, E. H., Erikson, J. M., & Kivnick, H. Q. (1986). *Vital involvement in old age*. New York: W. W. Norton & Company.

Erikson, E. H., & Erikson, J. M. (1997). *The life cycle completed*. New York: Norton.

Etherington, D., Lewis, S., & Mark, A.. (2008). *United Kingdom: report on emerging themes from the interviews*. Deliverable EU-project Quality, Utrecht: Utrecht University. Retrieved August 3rd 2010, from: http://eprints.mdx.ac/3758/1/United_Kingdom_-_report_on_emerging_themes_from_the_intereviews.pdf.

Ethnic Communities Oral History Project. (1993). *Asian voices*. London: author.

Exquemelin, A. O. (1678/1969). *The Buccaneers of America* (A. Brown, Trans). Harmondsworth, UK: Penguin.

Fanon, F. (1986). *Black skin, white masks*. London: Pluto.

Feldman, D. B., & Snyder, C. R. (2005). Hope and the meaningful life: Theoretical and empirical associations between goal-directed thinking and life meaning. *Journal of Social and Clinical Psychology, 24*(3), 401-421.

Fernandez-Armesto, F. (2000). *Civilizations*. London: Macmillan.

Fernandez-Armesto, F. (2001). *Truth: A history and a guide for the perplexed*. New York: Thomas Dunne/St Martin's Griffin.

Finke, J. (2003). *Meru – history*. Retrieved January 5, 2013, from http://www.bluegecko.org/kenya/tribes/meru/history.htm.

Flanders, J (2006). *Consuming passions. Leisure and pleasure in Victorian Britain*. London: Harper Collins.

Fleer, J., Hoekstra, H. J., Sleijfer, D. T., Tuiman, M. A., & Hoekstra-Weebers, J. E. (2006). The role of meaning in the prediction of psychosocial well-being of testicular cancer survivors. *Quality of Life Research, 15*, 705-717.

Fisch, K. (2008). *Did you know*. Video. Retrieved March 14, 2013, from *www.youtube.com/watch?v=5o9nmUB2qls*

Foner, P.S. (1965). *The AFL in the progressive era 1910-1915. History of the labor movement in the United States Volume 5*. New York: International Publishers.

Foner, P.S. (1980). *The International Workers of the World 1905-1917. History of the labor movement in the United States Volume 4*. New York: International Publishers.

Forbush, W. B. (1928). *Myths and legends of Greece and Rome*. Philadelphia: The John C. Winston Company.

Francis-Connolly, E. (1998). It Never Ends: Mothering as a Lifetime Occupation.

Scandinavian Journal of Occupational Therapy. 5: 149-155.

Frank, A. (1995). *The wounded storyteller. Body, illness, and ethics.* Chicago: The University of Chicago.

Frank, G. (1992). Opening feminist histories of occupational therapy. *American Journal of Occupational Therapy*, *46*(11), 988-999.

Frank, G., & Zemke, R. (2008). Occupational therapy foundations for political engagement and social transformation. In: N. Pollard, D. Sakellariou, & F. Kronenberg (Eds.) *A political practice of occupational therapy* (pp. 111-136). Edinburgh: Elsevier Science.

Frankl, V. E. (1966). Self-Transcendence as a Human Phenomenon. *Journal of Humanistic Psychology 6*, 97-106.

Frankl, V. E. (1969). *The doctor and the soul, from psychotherapy to logotherapy.* London: Souvenir Press.

Frankl, V. E. (1978). *The unheard cry for meaning.* New York: Touchstone.

Frankl, V. E. (1992). *Man's search for meaning: An introduction to logotherapy* (4th ed.). Boston, MA: Beacon Press.

Frankl, V. E. (1997). *Recollections: An autobiography* (Trans. J. Fabry). London: Plenum.

Frankl, V. E. (2000). *Man's ultimate search for meaning.* Cambridge, MA: Perseus.

Frumkin, H., Hess,J., Luber,G., Malilay, J., & McGeehin, M. (2008). Climate change: The public health response. *American Journal of Public Health.* (98):435-445.

Fryer, P. (1987) *Staying power. The history of Black people in Britain.* London: Pluto

Fuggle, R. F. (2001). *Lake Victoria: A case study of complex interrelationships.* Nairobi, Kenya: United Nations Environmental Programme.

Gardiner, M. (1985). *The other side of the counter.* Brighton, UK: QueenSpark.

Gatehouse. (1997). *Working lives, the experiences of 15 workers, from the 40's to the present day.* Manchester: Author.

Gauvain, M. (2001). *The social context of cognitive development.* New York: Guilford Press.

Gee, S., & Baillie, J. (1999). Happily ever after? An exploration of retirement expectations. *Educational Gerontologist, 25*(2), 109-128.

Gibbons, J. L., & Ashdown, B. K. (2006, August 30). A review of "Emerging adults in America: Coming of age in the 21st century" by Jeffrey Jensen Arnett and Jennifer Lynn Tanner (Eds.). *PsycCRITIQUES, 51*(35), Article 3.

Ginzbe rg, E., Ginzberg, S. W., Axelrad, S., & Herma, J. L. (1951). *Occupational choice: An approach to a general theory.* New York: Columbia University Press.

Goffman, E. (1978). *The presentation of self in everyday life.* Harmondsworth: Pelican.

Gomberg, P (2007). *How to make opportunity equal: Race and contributive justice.* Malden, MA: Blackwell.

Gordon, I. (1985). *It can happen.* Hackney, UK: Centerprise.

Gordon, J. (1983). Is the existence of God relevant to the meaning of life? *The Modern Schoolman, 60*, 227-246.

Gottfredson, L. S. (1996). Gottfredson's theory of circumscription and compromise. In D. Brown & L. Brooks (Eds), *Career choice and development* (pp 179-232). San Francisco, CA: Jossey Bass.

Graves, R. (1960). *The Greek myths: 1.* Harmondsworth: Pelican.

Greenspan, S., & Greenspan, N. T. (1985). *First feelings*. New York: Penguin Books.

Greenspan, S., & Lewis, N. B. (1999). *Building healthy minds*. New York: Penguin Books.

Grimshaw, D., Carroll, M., & Rubery, J. (2008). *Decent Work Country Report -United Kingdom.* International Labour Office Regional Office for Europe and Central Asia. Retrieved July 8th 2010, from http://www.ilo.int/public/english/region/eurpro/geneva/download/events/lisbon2009/wreports/dw_uk.pdf.

Hagerman, F. C., Fielding, R. A., Fiatarone, M. A., Gault, J. A., Kirkendall, D. T., Ragg, K. E., & Evans, W. J. (1996). A 20-yr. longitudinal study of Olympic oarsmen. *Medicine & Science in Sports & Exercise, 28*(9), 1150-1156.

Haidt, J. (2006). *The happiness hypothesis: Finding modern truth in ancient wisdom.* New York: Basic Books.

Hall, D. (1985). *Growing up in Ditchling*. Brighton, UK: QueenSpark.

Hamel, S., Leclerc, G., & Lefrancoise, R. (2003). A psychological outlook on the concept of transcendent actualization. *International Journal of Psychology and Religion, 13*(1), 3-15.

Hammell, K. W. (2004). Dimensions of meaning in the occupations of daily life. *Canadian Journal of Occupational Therapy, 71*(5), 296-305.

Hammell, K. W. (2007). Client-centred practice: Ethical obligation or professional obfuscation? *British Journal of Occupational Therapy*. 70(6) 264-6.

Hammell, K. W. (2008). Reflections on...well-being and occupational rights. *Canadian Journal of Occupational Therapy*. 75, 61-64.

Hammell, K. W. (2010). Contesting assumptions in occupational therapy. In M.Curtin, M. Molineaux & J. Supyk-Mellson (Eds), *Occupational therapy and physical dysfunction* (pp. 39-54). Edinburgh: Churchill Livingstone/Elsevier.

Handy, C. (2002). *The elephant and the flea: Reflections of a reluctant capitalist*. Boston, MA: Harvard Business School Press.

Hardin, G. (1991, Spring). Carrying capacity and quality of life. *The Social Contract*.

Harlow, L., Newcomb, M.D., & Bentler, P.M. (1986). Depression, self-derogation, substance use, and suicide ideation: Lack of purpose in life as a mediational factor. *Journal of Clinical Psychology*, 42(1) 5–21,

Harris, H. (1978). *Under oars.* Hackney, UK: Centerprise.

Hasselkus, B. R. (2002). *The meaning of every-day occupation*. Thorofare, NJ: Slack.

Havighurst, R. J. (1952). *Developmental tasks and education*. New York: David McKay.

Havighurst, R. J. (1971). *Developmental tasks and education* (3rd ed.). New York: Longman.

Havighurst, R. (1972). *Developmental tasks and education* (3rd ed.). New York: David McKay Company.

Havighurst, R. J. (1982). The world of work. In B. B. Wolman (Ed.), *Handbook of developmental psychology* (pp. 771-987). Englewood Cliffs, NJ: Prentice Hall.

Hawking, S. W. (1988). *A brief history of time: From the big bang to black holes*. New York: Bantam Books.

Hawking, S. W. (1994). *Black holes and baby universes and other essays*. New York: Bantam Books.

Hawking, S. W. (1996). Striving for excellence in the presence of disabilities. In R. Zemke & F. Clark (Eds.), *Occupational science: The evolving discipline* (pp. 27-30). Philadelphia: F. A. Davis.

Hayashi, A. (2002). Finding the voice of Japanese wilderness. *International Journal of Wilderness, 8*(2), 34-37.

Haylett, C. (2003). Culture, class and urban policy: reconsidering equality. *Antipode. 35*, 55 – 73.

Healey, B. (1980). *Hard times & easy terms.* Brighton, QueenSpark.

Heckhausen, J., & Schulz, R. (1993). Optimization by selection and compensation: Balancing primary and secondary control in life span development. *International Journal of Behavioral Development, 16,* 287-303.

Heckhausen, J. (1999). *Developmental regulation in adulthood: Age-normative and sociostructural constraints as adaptive challenges.* Cambridge, England: Cambridge University Press.

Heckhausen, J., Schulz, R., & Wrosch, C. (2010). A motivational theory of life-span development. *Psychological Review, 117*(1), 32-60.

Hergenhahn, B. R. (1997). *An introduction to the history of psychology.* Pacific Grove, CA: Brooks/Cole.

Hergenhahn, B. R. (2004). An introduction to the history of psychology (5th ed.). : Wadsworth Publishing.

Hibbert, C. (2001) *Queen Victoria: a personal history.* London: Da Capo.

Hicks, S. (1982) *Sparring for luck, autobiography of the East End boxer-poet.* London: Tower Hamlets Arts Project.

Higgs, J. & Titchen, A. (2001). Rethinking the practice-knowledge interface in an uncertain world: a model for practice development. *British Journal of Occupational Therapy.* 64(11), 526-533.

Hobsbawm, E. (1983). Introduction: inventing traditions. In E. Hobsbawm, & T. Ranger (Eds), *The invention of tradition* (pp. 1-14). Cambridge: Cambridge University Press.

Hocking, C. (1994). A model of interaction between objects, occupation, society, and culture. *Journal of Occupational Science, 1*(3), 28-45.

Hogg, M. A. (2001). A social identity theory of leadership. *Personality and Social Psychology Review, 5*(3), 184-200.

Hollick, B. (1992). *Pullman attendant.* Brighton, UK: QueenSpark.

Hoppes, S. (2005a). When a child dies the world should stop spinning: An autoethnography exploring the impact of family loss on occupation. *American Journal of Occupational Therapy, 59*(1), 78-87.

Hoppes, S. (2005b). Meanings and purposes of caring for a family member: An autoethno graphy. *American Journal of Occupational Therapy, 59*(3), 262-272.

Hornsey, M. J. (2008). Social identity theory and self-categorization theory: A historical review. *Social and personality Psychology Compass, 2/1*, 204-222.

Hughes, M. (2006). Affect, meaning and quality of life. *Social Forces, 85*(2), 611-629.

Hurd, J. P. (2004). Unto others: The evolution and psychology of unselfish behavior/ Darwin's cathedral [Book review]. *Christian Scholar's Review, 34*(1), 149-152.

Husk, K., Lovell, R., Cooper, C., & Garside, R. (2013), Participation in environmental enhancement and conservation activities for health and well-being in adults. *Cochrane database of systematic reviews 2013*. Issue 2. Art. No. CD010351. DOI. 10.1002/14651858.CD010351.

Ikiugu, M. N. (2001). The philosophy and culture of occupational therapy (Doctoral Dissertation, Texas Woman's University, 2001). *Dissertation Abstracts International, 62*(12B), 5678.

Ikiugu, M. N. (2004a). Instrumentalism in occupational therapy: An argument for a pragmatic conceptual model of practice. *International Journal of Psychosocial Rehabilitation, 8*, 109-117.

Ikiugu, M. N. (2004b). Instrumentalism in occupational therapy: A theoretical core for the pragmatic conceptual model of practice. *International Journal of Psychosocial Rehabilitation, 8*, 151-163.

Ikiugu, M. N. (2004c). Instrumentalism in occupational therapy: Guidelines for practice. *International Journal of Psychosocial Rehabilitation, 8*, 165-179.

Ikiugu, M. N. (2005). Meaningfulness of occupations as an occupational life trajectory attractor. *Journal of Occupational Science, 12*(3), 102-109

Ikiugu, M. N. (2007). *Psychosocial conceptual practice models in occupational therapy: Building adaptive capability*. St. Louis, MO: Mosby.

Ikiugu, M. N. (2008). *Occupational science in the service of Gaia: An essay describing a possible contribution of occupational scientists to the solution of prevailing global issues.* Baltimore, MD: PublishAmerica.

Ikiugu, M. N. (2010). The new occupational therapy paradigm: Implications for integration of the psychosocial core of occupational therapy in all clinical specialties. *Occupational Therapy in Mental Health, 26*(4), 343-353.

Ikiugu, M. N. (2011). Influencing social challenges through occupational performance. In F. Kronenberg, N. Pollard, & D. Sakellariou (Eds.), *Occupational therapies without borders* (pp. 113-122). London: Churchill Livingstone/Elsevier.

Ikiugu, M. N., Anderson, A., & Manas, D. (2008). The test-retest reliability of a battery of new occupational performance assessments. *International Journal of Therapy and Rehabilitation, 15*(12), 562-571.

Ikiugu, M. N., & McCollister, L. (2011). An occupation-based framework for changing human occupational behavior to address critical global issues. *International Journal of Professional Practice, 2*(4), 402-417.

Ikiugu, M. N., Pollard, N., Cross, A., Willer, M., Stockland, J., & Everson, J. (2012). Meaning-making through occupations and occupational roles: A heuristic study of worker-writer histories. *British Journal of Occupational Therapy, 75*, 289-295.

Ikiugu, M. N., & Rosso, H. M. (2005). Understanding the occupational human being as a complex, dynamical, adaptive system. *Occupational Therapy in Health Care, 19*(4), 43-65. Ikiugu, M. N., & Schultz, S. (2006). An argument for pragmatism as a foundational philosophy of occupational therapy. *Canadian Journal of Occupational Therapy, 73*(2), 86-97

Ikiugu, M. N., Westerfield, M. A., Lien, J. M., Theisen, E. R., Cerny, S. L., & Nissen,

R. M. (In press). Empowering people to change occupational behaviours to address critical global issues. *Canadian Journal of Occupational Therapy.*

Illich, I. (1980). *The right to useful unemployment.* London: Marion Boyars.

Irigaray, L. (1993). *Je, tu, nous, toward a culture of difference.* London: Routledge.

Ivanov, A. (2011, September). From London riots to Arab spring. Measuring social exclusion is a first step to address it. Voices from Eurasia [Online version]. United Nations Development Program in Europe and CIS. Retrieved January 2nd, 2013, from www.europeandcis.undp.org/blog/2011/09/05/from-london-riots-to-arab-spring/.

Iwasaki, Y. (2007). Leisure and quality of life in an international and multicultural context: What are major pathways linking leisure to quality of life? *Social Indicators Research, 82*, 233-264.

Jackson, J. (1995). Sexual orientation: its relevance to occupational science and the practice of occupational therapy. *American Journal of Occupational Therapy.* 49(7), **669-679**

Jackson, J., Carlson, M., Mandel, D., Zemke, R., & Clark, F. (1998). Occupation in lifestyle redesign: The well elderly study occupational therapy program. *American Journal of Occupational Therapy, 52*, 326-336.

Jahoda, M. (1981). Work, employment, and unemployment: Values, theories, and approaches in social research. *American Psychologist, 36*(2), 184-191.

James, L. (2006). *The middle class, a history.* London: Little, Brown.

James,W. (1981). *Pragmatism.* Indianapolis, Cambridge: Hackett.

Jamuhuri Team. (2012, July 4). The forgotten MAU MAU field marshal, Musa Mwariama. *Jamuhuri Magazine.* Retrieved January 5, 2013, from http://jamhurimagazine.com/index.php/icon/3550-the-forgotten-mau-mau-field-marshal-musa-mwariama.html.

Jewish Reconstructionists Federation. (2013). Who is a reconstructionist Jew? [Electronic version]. *Jewish Virtual Library.* Retrieved January 11th 2013, from http://www.jewishvirtuallibrary.org/jsource/Judaism/reconstruction.html.

Jewison, N. (Director). (1971). *Fiddler on the roof* [Motion picture]. Available from Cartier Productions, Hollywood, USA.

Jim, H. S., & Andersen, B. L. (2007). Meaning in life mediates the relationship between social and physical functioning and distress in cancer survivors. *British Journal of Health Psychology, 12*, 363-381.

Jones, A. (1995). *Larousse dictionary of world folklore.* Edinburgh: Larousse.

Jones, R.G. (1984). *Groundwork of Christian ethics.* London: Epworth.

Jung, C. G. (1971). *Psychological types.* Princeton, New Jersey: Princeton University Press.

Jung, C. G. (1983/1953). *The collected works of C. G. Jung.* Princeton: Princeton University Press.

Jung, C. G. (1985, November 8). Integrating anima and animus. *Therapy Weekly,* 15.

Kanu, M. A. (n.d.). *The indispensability of the basic social values in African traditions: A philosophical appraisal.* Found at http://www.ajol.info/index.php/og/article/viewFiles/57930/46296.

Kaplan, A.M. & Haenlein, M (2010). Users of the world, unite! The challenges and opportunities of Social Media. *Business Horizons* (53), 59-68

Kazez, J. (2007). *The weight of things: philosophy and the good life.* Oxford: Blackwell.

Kelley, A. C. (1988). Economic consequences of population change in the third world. *Journal of Economic Literature*, 26, 1685-1728.

Kelly, J. R., & Kelly, J. R. (1994). Multiple dimensions of meaning in the domains of work, family, and leisure [Electronic version]. *Journal of Leisure Research, 26*(3), 1-15. Retrieved April 25, 2008, from http://proquest.umi.com/pqdweb?index=14&sid=4&srchmode=1&vinst=PROD&fmt=3$s...

Kennedy, G. (1996). John Dewey: Introduction. In M. H. Fisch (Ed.), *Classic American philosophers* (pp. 327-335). New York: Fordham University Press.

Keynes, J. M. (1936/2003). *The general theory of employment, interest, and money.* Retrieved July 8th 2010, from http://cas.umkc.edu/ECON/economics/Kregel/645/Winter2008/Keynes,%2520John2520Maynard%2520 %2520General%2520Theory%2520of%2520Employment%2520(1936).pdf.

Kielhofner, G. (2008). *Model of human occupation: Theory and application* (4th ed.). Philadelphia: Lippincott Williams & Wilkins.

Kielhofner, G. (2009). *Conceptual foundations of occupational therapy practice* (4th ed.). Philadelphia: F. A. Davis.

King, M. L. (2000). *The autobiography of Martin Luther King* (Clayborne Crayson, Ed.) London: Abacus.

Kiogora, D. S., Njoka, E. M., Khaemba, J. M., Komwihangilo, D. M., & Max, R. A. (2011).

Anthropogenic factors influencing the ruminant food chain in Lake Victorian Basin. *International Journal of Professional Practice, 2*(4), 321-330.

Kiragu, S. (2011). Adaptation to a Changing Climate: Capacities of Kenya's Dryland Women. In A. Daniel, K. Fink, L. Kroeker, J. Schütze (eds.) *BIGSAS Working Papers 1/2011: Women's Life Worlds 'In-Between'*. (pp41-57). Bayreuth: Universitat Bayreuth.

Kissane, D.W. (2000). Distress, demoralisation and depression in palliative care. *Current Therapetics.* 6, 14-9

Krasko, G. L. (1997). Viktor Frankl: The prophet of meaning [Electronic version]. *Journals des Viktor-Frankl-Instituts, 5*(1), p. 82. Retrieved February 21, 2008, from http://stuff.mit.edu/people/gkrasko/Frankl.html.

Kreamer, A. (2013). The formula for creating happiness at work. *Fast Company*. Retrieved on January 7, 2013, from http://www.fastcompany.com/print/3003982.

Kronenberg, F., & Pollard, N. (2005). Overcoming occupational apartheid: A preliminary exploration of the political nature of occupational therapy. In F. Kronenberg, N. Pollard, & D. Sakellariou (Eds.), *Occupational therapy without borders. Learning from the spirit of survivors* (pp. 58-86). Edinburgh: Elsevier/Churchill Livingstone.

Kronenberg, F, Simo Algado, S and Pollard N (2005) (eds), *Occupational Therapy without borders -learning from the spirit of survivors*, Edinburgh, Elsevier Science.

Kronenberg F, Pollard N, Sakellariou D (eds) (2011) *Occupational therapies without borders (Volume 2).* Edinburgh, Elsevier Science.

Kuh, D., Hardy, R., Butterworth, S., Okell, L., Richards, M., Wadsworth, M., Sayer, A.

A. (2006). Developmental origins of midlife physical performance: Evidence from a British birth cohort. *American Journal of Epidemiology, 164*(2), 110-121.

Kumar, A. (2011). Bharatanatyam and identity making in the South Asian diaspora: Culture through the lens of occupation. *Journal of Occupational Science.* 18(1), 36-47

Lachman, M. E., & James, J. B. (1997). *Multiple paths of midlife development.* Chicago: Chicago University Press.

Lafargue, P. (1996 [1883]). *La droit a la pareses: refutation du Droit au travail de 1848.* Pantin: Le temps de Cerises.

Lai, J. C., Chong, A. M., Siu, O. T., Evans, P., Chan, C. L., & Ho, R. T. (2010). Humor attenuates the cortisol awakening response in healthy older men. *Biological Psychology, 84*, 375-380.

Lang, A. (1892). (Ed.) *The green fairy book.* On line. Available at www.childrensnursery.org.uk/fairy.../green-fairy-book.html. Last accessed 3.9.09.

Law, M., Polatajko, H., Baptiste, S., & Townsend, E. (2002). Core concepts of occupational therapy. In E. Townsend (Ed), *Enabling occupation: an occupational therapy* perspective (pp. 29-56). Ottawa, ON: Canadian Association of Occupational Therapists.

Law, M. (2002). Participation in the occupations of everyday life. *American Journal of Occupational Therapy, 56*, 640-649.

Lentin, P. (2002): The Human Spirit and Occupation: Surviving and Creating a Life. *Journal of Occupational Science*, 9:3, 143-152

Leprince De Beaumont, J. M. (2009/1783). *Beauty and the Beast.* On line. Available at http://www.pitt.edu/~dash/folk**text**s.html. Last accessed 11.09.09.

Lesunyane, A. (2010). Psychiatry and mental health in Africa: the vital role of occupational therapy. In V. Alers & R Crouch (eds.) *Occupational Therapy: an African perspective.* (pp 286-303). Johannesburg: Sarah Shorten.

Letablier, M., Luci, A., Math, A., & Thévenon, O. (2009) *The costs of raising children and the effectiveness of policies to support parenthood in European countries: a Literature Review.* European Commission, Directorate-General for Employment, Social Affairs and Equal Opportunities, Unit for Social and Demographic Analysis. Retrieved 11.3.2013 from http://hal.archives- ouvertes.fr/docs/00/40/88/99/PDF/EU_Report_Cost_of_children_Final_11-05-2009.pdf

Levinson, D. J. (1978). *The seasons in a man's life.* New York: Knopf.

Levinson, D. J., & Levinson, J. D. (1996). *Seasons of a woman's life.* New York: Alfred A. Knopf.

Lewchanin, S., & Zubrod, L. A. (2001). Choices in life: A clinical tool for facilitating midlife review. *Journal of Adult Development, 8*(3), 193-196.

Lewis, S., Tarrier, N., Haddock, G., Bentall, R., Kinderman, P., Kingdon, D., and Dunn, G. (2002). Randomised controlled trial of cognitive-behavioural therapy in early schizophrenia: Acute-phase outcomes. *British Journal of Psychiatry, 181*(Suppl. 43), s91-s97.

Lloyd, A. E. (1969). *Folk song in England.* London: Panther.

Lohan, M., Cruise, S., O'Halloran, P., Alderdice, F., & Hyde, A. (2010). Adolescent

men's attitudes in relation to pregnancy and pregnancy outcomes: a systematic review of the literature from 1980–2009. *Journal of Adolescent Healt.h* 47, 327–345
Lord, W. (1958). *A night to remember.* London: Corgi.
Luthuli, A. (1963). *Let my people* go. London: Fontana.
Lydon, J. (1998). *The making of Ireland. From ancient times to the present.* London: Routledge.
Lyons, M., & Tarrier, A. (2004). *Espejos y ventanas/Mirrors and Windows.* Philadephia: New City Community Press.
Maathai, W. (2010). *Spiritual values for healing ourselves and the world: Replenishing the earth.* New York: Doubleday.
McAdams, D. P. (2006). The problem of narrative coherence. *Journal of Constructivist Psychology, 19*, 109-125.
McFarland, S., & Mathews, M. (2005). Who cares about human rights? *Political Psychology, 26*(3), 365-385.
McKelvey, B. (1997). *Organization positivism: Separating myth from reality.* The Anderson School at the University of California at Los Angeles. Paper presented at the Macro Organizational Behavior Society Meeting.
MacKillop, J. (2004). "Oisín". *A Dictionary of Celtic Mythology.* Retrieved September 03, 2009 from Encyclopedia.com: http://www.encyclopedia.com/doc/1O70-Oisn.html.
McNamee, S. J. (2007). The social construction of life meaning: The 2007 North Carolina Sociological Association presidential address [Electronic version]. *Sociation Today, 5*(2), 1-15. Retrieved April 25, 2008, from http://www.ncsociology.org/sociationtoday/v52/steve.htm.
Magee, B. (1998). *The story of thought: The essential guide to the history of Western philosophy.* New York: D. K. Publishing.
Mahler, M. S., Pine, F., & Bergman, A. (1975). *The psychological birth of the human infant* .New York: Basic Books.
Mair, L. (1962). *Primitive government.* Harmondsworth: Pelican.
Mandela, N. (1994). *Long walk to freedom.* London: Abacus.
Manthorpe, J., Hussein, S., Stevens, M. & Moriarty, J. (2012). User and Carer Experiences of International Social Care Workers in England: Listening to their Accounts of Choice and Control. *Australian Social Work, 65*(4), 442-456.
Manville, S. (1989). *Everything seems smaller.* Brighton, UK: QueenSpark.
Manville, S. (1994). *Our small corner.* Brighton, UK: QueenSpark.
Markale, J (1977). *Histoire secrete de la Bretagne.* Paris: Albin Michel
Marr, A. (2007). *The history of modern Britain.* London: Macmillan.
Marr, A. (2009). *The making of modern Britain.* London: Macmillan.
Marsh, P., Bradley, S., Love, C., Alexander, P., & Norham, R. (2007). *Belonging.* Oxford, UK: Social Issues Research Center
Marshall, J. (1984). *The King's own Yorkshireman.* Barnsley, UK: Yorkshire Arts Circus.
Martin, R. (2011, October 23). Why current population growth is costing us the earth [On-line version]. The Guardian. Retrieved July 30, 2012, from http://www.

guardian.co.uk/environment/2011/oct/23/why-population-growth-costs-the-ear...
Mascaro, N., & Rosen, D. H. (2005). Existential meaning's role in the enhancement of hope and prevention of depressive symptoms. *Journal of Personality, 73*(4), 985-1013.
Maslow, A. H. (1970). *Motivation and personality* (2nd ed.). New York: Harper & Row.
Maslow, A. H. (1971). *The further reaches of human nature.* Harmondsworth: Penguin.
Mason, E. (1998). *A working man, a century of Hove memories.* Brighton, UK: QueenSpark.
Mason, M. (2002). *Incurably human.* London: wORking Press.
Masterson, O. (1986). *The circle of life.* Brighton, UK: QueenSpark.
Mattingly, C. (1998). *Healing dramas and clinical plots.* Cambridge: Cambridge University Press.
Matuska, K. M. & Christiansen, C. H. (2008). A proposed model of lifestyle balance, *Journal of Occupational Science*, 15:1, 9-19
Max-Neef, M. (1991). *Human scale development conception, application and further reflections.* New York: The Apex Press.
Max-Neef, M. (2010). The world on a collision course and the need for a new economy. *AMBIO, 39*, 200-210.
Mayer, K. U. (2002). *The sociology of the life course and life span psychology – diverging or converging pathways?* Unpublished Manuscript.
Mayer, K. U. (2000). Promises fulfilled? A review of twenty years of life course research. *Archives Europeennes de Sociologie, XLI*(2), 259-282.
Maynard, S. S., & Kleiber, D. A. (2005). Using leisure services to build social capital in later life: Classical traditions, contemporary realities, and emerging possibilities. *Journal of Leisure Research, 37*(4), 475-493.
Mead, G.H. (1932). *The philosophy of the present.* Chicago: Open Court.
Metz, T. (2007). The meaning of life [Electronic version]. *Stanford Encyclopedia of Philosophy*. Retrieved March 13 2008, from http://plato.stanford.edu/entries/life-meaning/.
Meyer, C. (2010). Developing services where there was no infrastructure. In V. Alers & R Crouch (eds.) *Occupational Therapy: an African perspective.* (pp 330-339). Johannesburg: Sarah Shorten.
Michaelson, C. (2007). Work and the most terrible life. *Journal of Business Ethics, 77*, 335-345.
Millbanks, C. (1986). *My way of living, twenty five years on.* Manchester: Gatehouse.
Mindell, A. (1982). *Dreambody.* Boston, MA: Sigo Press.
Mindell, A. (1995). *Sitting in the fire: Large group transformation using conflict and diversity.* Portland, OR: Lao Tse Press.
Mindell, A. (2001). *Working with the dreaming body.* Portland, OR: Lao Tse Press.
Mindell, A. (2002). *The deep democracy of open forums: Practical steps to conflict prevention and resolution for the family, workplace, and world.* Newburyport, MA: Hampton Roads Publishing Company.
Moav, O. (2004). Cheap children and the persistence of poverty. *The Economic Journal*, 115, 88-110.
Monaf, N. (1994). *New home, hard work.* Manchester: Gatehouse.

Morel, C.M. & E. Mossialos, (2010). Stoking the antibiotic pipeline. *British Medical Journal.* 340 doi: http://dx.doi.org/10.1136/bmj.c2115

Morita, T. (2004). Differences in physician-reported practice in palliative sedation therapy. *Supportive Care In Cancer.* 12 (8), 584-592

Morley, D., Worpole, K., & Pollard, N. (2009). Class identity and the republics of letters. In D. Morley, & K. Worpole. (Eds), *The republic of letters* (2nd ed.) (pp. 223-244. Philadelphia: New Cities Community Press/Syracuse University Press.

Morojele, N.K., & Brook, J.S. (2004) Sociodemographic, sociocultural, and individual predictors of reported feelings of meaninglessness among South African adolescents. *Psychological Reports*: Volume 95, 1271-1278

Mosey, A. C. (1996). *Applied scientific inquiry in the health professions: An epistemological orientation* (2nd ed.). Bethesda, MD: AOTA Press.

Moss, F. (1986). *City pit.* Bristol, UK: Bristol Broadsides.

Mottainai Campaign Office. (2012). *About Mottainai campaign.* Found at http://mottainai.info/english/.

Muckle, W. (1981). *No regrets.* Newcastle upon Tyne, UK: People's Publications.

Murphy, R. F. (2001). *The body silent: The different world of the disabled.* New York: W. W. Norton & Company.

Nagel, T. (1986). *The view from nowhere.* Oxford: Oxford University Press.

Nassos, G. P. (n.d.). *A sustainable environment: Our obligation to protect God's gift.* Available at http://www.georgepnassos.com/Goerge_P_Nassos/Articles_files/Exceeding_the_Carrying. National Academy of Sciences. (1997). *Preparing for the 21st century: The environment and the human nature* [On-line Version]. Retrieved June 13, 2012, from http://www.nas.edu/21st/environment/environment.html.

National Records of Scotland (2011), *Life Expectancy for areas in Scotland, 2008-2010.* Edinburgh: author.

Neville-Jan, A. (2004). Selling your soul to the devil: an autoethnography of pain, pleasure and the quest for a child. *Disability and Society*, 19(2) 113-127.

Newby, H (1977). *The deferential worker.* London: Allen Lane.

Noakes D (1980a) *The town beehive – a young girl's lot, Brighton 1910-1934.* Brighton, QueenSpark

Noakes D (1980b) *Faded rainbow, our married years.* Brighton, QueenSpark

Noakes, G. (1977). *To be a farmer's boy.* Brighton, UK: QueenSpark.

Noble, E. M. (1984). *Jamaica airman, a black airman in Britain, 1943 and after.* London: New Beacon.

Nozick, R. (1981). *Philosophical explanations.* Oxford: Clarendon Press

Nozick, R. (1989). *The examined life.* New York: Simon and Schuster

Pinel, P. (1962). *A Treatise on Insanity.* (Davis, D.D., Trans.). New York: Hafner Publishing Company.

Padfield, D. (Ed). (1999). *Hidden lives, stories from the East End by the people of 42 Balaam Street.* London/Kelso Eastside Community Heritage: Curlew Productions.

Palmer, R. (1988). *The sound of history: Songs and social comment.* London: Pimlico.

Pargament, K. I. (2008). The sacred character of community life. *American Journal of*

Community Psychology, 41, 22-34.

Parsons, J. (1995). *Jobs for life*. Brighton, UK: QueenSpark.

Passmore, A. (2003). The occupation of leisure: Three typologies and their influence on mental health in adolescence. *Occupational Therapy Journal of Rehabilitation, 23*(2) 76-83.

Paul, A. (1981). *Hard work and no consideration, 51 years as a carpenter-joiner 1917-1968*. Brighton, UK: QueenSpark.

Paul, E. F., Miller, F. D., & Paul, J. (Eds.). (1997). *Self-interest*. New York: Cambridge University Press.

Paul, K. I., Geithner, E., & Moser, K. (2009): Latent deprivation among people who are employed, unemployed, or out of the labor force. *The Journal of Psychology: Interdisciplinary and Applied, 143*(5), 477-491.

Pearsall, R. (1983). *The worm in the bud, the world of Victorian sexuality*. Harmondsworth: Penguin.

Peirce, C. S. (1955). The fixation of belief. In J. Buchler (Ed.), *Philosophical writings of Peirce* (pp. 5-22). New York: Dover.

Percy, T. (1966). (Ed). *Reliques of ancient English poetry, volume 1* (pp. xiii-xcvii). New York: Dover.

Perkins, D. F. (2007). *Adolescence: Developmental tasks*. University of Florida IFAS Extension.

Peterson, J. B. (2000). *The pragmatics of meaning*. Retrieved March 3, 2008, from http://www.semioticon.com/frontline/jordan_b.htm.

Piaget, J. (1999/1950). *The psychology of intelligence*. New York: Routledge.

Pickens, N. D., & Pizur-Barnekow, K. (2009). Co-occupation: Extending the dialogue. *Journal of Occupational Science, 16*(3), 151-156.

Peirce, C. S. (1955). The fixation of belief. In J. Buchler, (Ed.), *Philosophical writings of Peirce* (pp. 5-22). New York: Dover Publications.

Piper, R. (1995) *Take him away*. Brighton, QueenSpark.

Pollard, N., & Walsh, S. (2000). Occupational therapy, gender and mental health: an inclusive perspective? *British Journal of Occupational Therapy 63* (9) 425-431.

Pollard, N. (2006). Is dying an occupation? *Journal of Occupational Science. 13*(2), 149-152.

Pollard N. (2010) Occupational narratives, community publishing and worker writing groups: Sustaining stories from the margins. *Groupwork*. 20(1) 9-33.

Pollard N, Kronenberg F, Sakellariou D. (2008). A political practice of occupational therapy. In N. Pollard, D. Sakellariou, F. Kronenberg (eds), *A political practice of occupational therapy*, (pp.3-20) Edinburgh, Elsevier Science.

Pollard N, Sakellariou D, Kronenberg F (2008) (eds), *A political practice of occupational therapy*, Edinburgh, Elsevier Science.

Pollard, N., & Sakellariou, D. (2012). Introduction. In N. Pollard & D. Sakellariou (Eds.), *Politics of occupation-centered practice: Reflections on occupational engagement across cultures*. West Sussex, UK: Wiley-Blackwell.

Pollard N, Smart P (2012) Making writing accessible to all: The Federation of Worker Writers and Community Publishers and TheFED. In P Mathieu, S Parks &

T Rousculp (eds) *Circulating communities: The tactics and strategies of community publishing.* Lanham MA: Lexington Books, pp21-34.

Poulsen, C. (1988). *Scenes from a Stepney youth.* London: Tower Hamlets Arts Project.

Price, P., & Stephenson, S. M. (2009). Learning to promote occupational development through co-occupation. *Journal of Occupational Science, 16*(3), 180-186.

Primorac, M. (2011, September 12). Income inequality: F& D spotlights widening gap between rich and poor [Online Version]. *IMF Survey Magazine: In the News.* Retrieved August 8, 2012, from http://www.imf.org/external/pubs/ft/survey/so/2011/NEW091211A.htm.

Pryor, F. (2004). *Britain B.C. Life in Britain and Ireland before the Romans.* London: Harper Perennial.

Putnam, R. (1995). Bowling alone: America's declining social capital. *Journal ofDemocracy, 6*(1), 65-78.

Putnam, R. D. (2000). *Bowling alone, the collapse and revival ofAmerican community.* New York: Simon and Schuster

Pytell, T. (2000).The missing pieces of the puzzle: A reflection on the odd career of Viktor Frankl. *Journal of Contemporary History, 35*(2), 281-306.

Pytell, T. (2001). The genesis of Viktor Frankl's third Viennese school of psychotherapy. *Psychoanalytic Review, 88,* 312–334.

Pytell, T. (2003). Redeeming the unredeemable: Auschwitz and 'Man's search for meaning'. *Holocaust and Genocide Studies.* 17(1), 89-113.

Pytell, T. (2007). Extreme experience, psychological insight, and holocaust perception: Reflections on Bettelheim and Frankl. *Psychoanalytic Psychology, 24*(4), 641–657.

Quinn, P. (2000). How Christianity secures life's meanings. In J. Runzo & N. Martin (Eds.), *The meaning of life in the world religions* (pp. 53-68). Oxford: Oneworld Publications.

Ragon, M. (1986). *Histoire de la litterature proletarienne de langue Française.* Paris: Albin Michel.

Rebeiro-Gruhl, K. L. (2009). The politics of practice: strategies to secure our occupational claim and to address occupational injustice *New Zealand Journal of Occupational Therapy.* 56(1): 19-26.

Redfield, J. (1994). *The Celestine prophecy, an adventure.* London, Bantam.

Reilly, M. (1962). Occupational therapy can be one of the great ideas of 20th century medicine. *American Journal of Occupational Therapy, 16,* 1–9.

Reker, G. T. (n.d.). Life attitude profile-revises (LAP-R). n.p.: Author

Resnick, M. (2007). *All I really need to know (about creative thinking) I learned (by studying how children learn) in kindergarten.* On line. Available: www.media.mit.edu/~mres/papers/kindergarten-learning-approach.pdf.

Reynolds, P., & Cronin, A. (2005). Aging. In A. Cronin & M. B. Mandich (Eds.), *Human development & performance throughout the lifespan* (pp. 306-331). Clifton Park, NY: Thomson Delmar Learning.

Ricoeur , P. (1980). Narrative time. *Critical Inquiry,* 7(1), 169-190.

Rosenberg, M. (1979). *Conceiving the self.* Malabar, FL: Robert E. Krieger.

Ross, E. (1984). *Tales of the rails.* Bristol, UK: Bristol Broadsides.

Rowe, D. (2003). *Depression, the way out of your prison.* London: Routledge.

Rowe, J. W., & Kahn, R. L. (1997). Successful aging. *The gerontologist, 37*(4), 433-440.

Rowland, C. (1988). *Radical Christianity.* Cambridge: Polity Press.

Rowles, G. (2008). Place in occupational science: A life course perspective on the role of environmental context in the quest of meaning. *Journal of Occupational Science, 15*(3), 127-135.

Royce, J. (1964). *The encapsulated man: An interdisciplinary essay on the search for meaning.* Princeton, NJ: D. Van Nostrand Company.

Russell, B. (1961). *History of Western philosophy.* London: Routledge.

Russell, D. (1997). *Popular music in England 1840-1914* (2nd edition). Manchester: Manchester University Press.

Russell, H. (n.d.). *Ageing well: Older adult computer learners.* University of Technology, Sydney, Australia. Retrieved January 10, 2012, from http://www.aare.edu.au/04pap/rus04241.pdf.

Sakellariou, D., & Pollard, N. (2008). Three sites of conflict and co-operation: class, gender and sexuality. In N. Pollard, D. Sakellariou & F. Kronenberg (Eds.), *A Political Practice of Occupational Therapy* (pp 69-89). Oxford: Elsevier Science.

Sakellariou, D., & Pollard, N. (2012). Narratives and truths. In N. Pollard & D. Sakellariou (Eds.), *Politics of Occupation-Centred Practice* (pp.). Oxford: Wiley, (In press).

Salmela-Aro, K., Aunola, K., & Nurmi, J. E. (2005). *Emerging adulthood and transition to work life.* Proceedings of the International Symposium on Youth and Work Culture on May 30-31, 2005, at Espoo Finnish Institute of Occupational Health

Salmon, N. (2006) The waiting place: A caregiver's narrative. *Australian Occupational Therapy Journal*, 53, 181-187.

Sames, K. (2009). *Documenting occupational therapy practice* (2nd Ed.). Upper Saddle River, NJ: Prentice Hall.

Schama, S. (1995). *Landscape and Memory.* London: HarperCollins.

Scharf, M., Mayseless, O., & Kivenson-Baron, I. (2004). Adolescents' attachment representations and developmental tasks in emerging adulthood. *Developmental Psychology, 40*(3), 430-444.

Schemm, R. L., & Gitlin, L. N. (1993). A model to promote activity competence in elders. *American Journal of Occupational Therapy, 47*, 147-153.

Schkade, J., & Schultz, S. (1992). Occupational adaptation: Toward a holistic approach to contemporary practice, Part I. *American Journal of Occupational Therapy, 46*, 829-837.

Schmidtz, D. (2001). The meaning of life. In L. Rouner (Ed.), *Boston University studies in philosophy and religion, volume 22; If I should die: Life, death, and immortality* (pp. 170-188). Notre Dame: University of Notre Dame Press.

Schultz, S., & Schkade, J. (1992). Occupational adaptation: Toward a holistic approach to contemporary practice, part 2. *American Journal of Occupational Therapy, 46*, 917-926.

Schwartz, S. J., Cote, J. E., & Arnett, J. J. (2005). Identity and agency in emerging adulthood: Two developmental routes in the individualization process. *Youth &*

Society, 37(2), 201-228.

Scott, W. (1987). *To a farmer born.* Bristol, UK: Bristol Broadsides.

Segal, R. (2005). Occupations and identity in the life of a primary caregiving father. *Journal of Occupational Science.* 12:2, 82-90

Seibers, T. (2008). *Disability theory.* Ann Arbor, MI: University of Michigan Press.

Semenza, J.C., Hall, D.E., Wilson, D.J., Bontempo, B.D., Sailor, D.J., & George, L.A. (2008). Public perception of climate change voluntary mitigation and barriers to behavior change. *American Journal of Preventative Medicine.* 35(5):479–487)

Sennett, R. & Cobb, J. (1972). *The hidden injuries of class.* New York: Alfred Knopf.

Serge, V. (1968). *The case of Comrade Tulayev.* Harmondsworth, UK: Penguin.

Seymour, W. (2002) Time and the body: Re-embodying time in disability. *Journal of Occupational Science.* 9(3), 135-142.

Shank, K. H., & Cutchin, M. P. (2010). Transactional occupations of older women aging-in-place: Negotiating change and meaning. *Journal of Occupational Science.* 17(1), 4-13

Shannon, C. S., & Bourque, D. (2005). Overlooked and underutilized: The critical role of leisure interventions in facilitating social support throughout breast cancer treatment and recovery. *Social Work in Health Care, 42*(1), 73-92.

Shaw, K., & Cronin, A. (2005). Adulthood. In A. Cronin & M. B. Mandich (Eds.), *Human development & performance throughout the lifespan* (pp. 284-305). Clifton Park, NY: Thomson Delmar Learning.

Sherrer, N. (n.d.). *Probing the relationship between Native Americans and ecology.* University of Alabama, Birmingham, Alabama.

Shordike, A., O'Brien, S.P., Marshall, (2011). From altruism to participation: bridging academia and borderlands. In F. Kronenberg, N. Pollard, & D. Sakellariou (Eds.), *Occupational therapies without borders* (pp. 329-338). London: Churchill Livingstone/ Elsevier.

Simo, S. (2011). Universities and the global change: inclusive communities, gardening and citizenship. In F. Kronenberg, N. Pollard, & D. Sakellariou (Eds.), *Occupational therapies without borders* (pp. 357-365). London: Churchill Livingstone/Elsevier.

Simpson, J. A., Collins, A., Tran, S., & Haydon, K. C. (2007). Attachment and the experience and expression of emotions in romantic relationships: A developmental perspective. *Journal of Personality and Social Psychology, 92*(2), 355-367.

Sinclair, K. (2007) Exploring the facets of clinical reasoning. In J. Creek & A Lawson-Porter (Eds.), *Contemporary issues in occupational therapy* (pp. 143-160). Oxford: Blackwell.

Sipsma, H., Brooks Biello, K.,Cole-Lewis, H., & Kerhsaw, T. (2010). Like father, like son: the intergenerational cycle of adolescent fatherhood. *American Journal of Public Health.* 100, 517–524.

Sitzia, L., & Thickett, A. (2002). *Seeking the enemy.* London: wORking press.

Smith, A, (1999). *The wealth of nations, books I-III.* Harmondsworth, UK: Penguin.

Smith, E. (1992). *Little Ethel Smith, her story told by herself.* Brighton, UK: QueenSpark.

Smith, J. Z. (1980). The bare facts of ritual. *History of Religions, 20*(1/2), 112-127.

Snyder, S. L., & Mitchell, D. T. (2006). *Cultural locations of disability.* Chicago: University of Chicago.

Southwick, S. M., Gilmartin, R., McDonough, P., & Morrissey, P. (2006). Logotherapy as an adjunctive treatment for chronic combat-related PTSD: A meaning-based intervention. *American Journal of Psychotherapy, 60*(2), 161-174.

Steer, A. (1994). *Brighton boy, a fifties childhood.* Brighton, UK: QueenSpark.

Steeves, H. L. (2008). Commodifying Africa on U.S. Network Reality Television. *Communication, Culture & Critique, 1*, 416–446.

Stets, J. E., & Burke, P. J. (2000). Identity theory and social identity theory. *Social Psychology Quarterly, 63*(3), 224-237.

Stevens-Long, J., & Commons, M. (1992). *Adult life* (4th ed.). Mountainview, CA: Mayfield.

Stoffel, V. C. (2013). Opportunities for occupational therapy behavioral health: A call to action. *American Journal of Occupational Therapy, 67*, 140-145.

Stolle, D., & Hooghe, M. (2004). Inaccurate, exceptional, one-sided or irrelevant? The debate about the alleged decline of social capital and civic engagement in western societies. *British Journal of Political Science, 35*, 149-167.

Strong, S. (1998). Meaningful work in supportive environments: Experiences with the recovery process. *American Journal of Occupational Therapy, 52*, 31-38.

Sullivan, S. E. (1999). The changing nature of careers: A review and research agenda. *Journal of Management, 25*(3), 457-484.

Sutherland, W.J., Bailey, M.J., Bainbridge, I.P., Brereton, T., Dick, J.T.A., Drewitt, J., Dulvy, N.K., et al (2008). Future novel threats and opportunities facing UK biodiversity identified by horizon scanning. *Journal of Applied Ecology*, 45(3) 821-833.

Suzuki, D. T. (1969). *An introduction to Zen Bhuddism.* London: Rider.

Tajfel, H. (1972). Social categorization: English manuscript of 'La categorization sociale'. In S. Moscovici (Ed.), *Introduction a la psychologie sociale* (Vol. 1, pp. 272-302). Paris, France: Larousse.

Tanner, J. L., & Arnett, J. J. (2009). The emergence of 'emerging adulthood': The new life stage between adolescence and young adulthood. In A. Furlong (Ed.), *Handbook of youth and young adulthood: New perspectives and agendas* (pp. 39-45). New York: Routledge.

Tatzer. V. C., van Nes, F., & Jonsson H. (2011) Understanding the Role of Occupation in Ageing: Four Life Stories of Older Viennese Women, *Journal of Occupational Science*, DOI:10.1080/14427591.2011.610774

Thew, M., Edwards, M., Baptiste, S., & Molineux, M. (Eds.) (2011). *Role emerging occupational therapy: Maximising occupation-focused practice.* Oxford: Wiley.

Thieme, A., Wallace, J., Olivier, P., & Meyer, T. D. (2012). *How can we support meaningful social relationships through digital design?* CHI, Austin, Texas.

Thomas, B., Dorling, D., & Davey Smith, G. (2010). An observational study of health inequalities in Britain: geographical divides returning to 1930s maxima by 2007. *British Medical Journal, 341*, c3639. doi:10.1136/bmj.c3639.

Thompson, P. (1993). Comment: 'I don't feel old': The significance of the search for meaning in later life. *International Journal of Geriatric Psychiatry, 8*, 685-692.

Thompson, P. (2007). The relationship of fatigue and meaning in life in breast cancer survivors. (Clinical report) [Electronic version]. *Oncology Nursing Forum*. Retrieved April 25, 2008, from http://www.encyclopedia.com/doc/1G1-166851131.html.

Tolstoy, L. (1960 /1886). The death of Ivan Ilyich. In R. Edmonds (tr.), *The Cossacks/ happy ever after/ The death of Ivan Ilyich.* Harmondsworth, UK: Penguin.

Tonner, L. (1995). *First time barmaid.* Manchester: Gatehouse.

Torres, C. (1973). *Revolutionary Priest.* Harmondsworth, UK: Penguin

Townsend, E. (1998). *Good intentions overruled: A critique of empowerment in the routine organization of mental health services.* Toronto, ON: University of Toronto Press.

Townsend, E., Langille, L., Ripley, D. (2003). Professional tensions in client-centered practice: Using institutional ethnography to generate understanding and transformation. *American Journal of Occupational Therapy, 57*, 17–28.

Trollope, J. (1994). *Britannia's daughters, women of the British empire.* Pimlico: London.

Trungpa, C. (1973). *Cutting through spiritual materialism.* Boulder, CO. Shambhala.

Tuke, S. (1964). *Description of the Retreat: An Institution near York for Insane persons of the Society of Friends Containing an Account of its Origin and Progress, The mode of Treatment, and a statement of Cases.* London: Dawsons of Pall Mall.

Tupe, D. (2013). Emerging theories. In B. A. Boyt-Schell, G. Gillen, & M. E. Scaffa (Eds), *Willard & Spackman's occupational therapy* (12th ed., pp. 553-562). Philadelphia: Lippincott Williams & Wilkins.

United Nations. (2011, May 3). World population to reach 10 billion by 2100 if fertility in all countries converges to replacement level [Online Version]. *New York Time.* Retrieved from http://foweb.unfpa.org/SWP2011/reports/Press_Release_WPP2010.pdf.

United Nations Environmental Program. (n.d.). *Human vulnerability to environmental change.* Found at http://www.unep.org/GEO/geo3/English/pdfs/Chapter3_ vulnerability.pdf.

United States Census Bureau. (2005, March 10). Census Bureau estimates number of children and adults in the States and Puerto Rico [Electronic version]. Retrieved July 16, 2010, from http://www.census.gov/newsroom/releases/archives/population/ c05-32.html.

United States Environmental Protection Agency. (1998). *Stay healthy in the sun.* Washington, D.C.: Author.

University of California San Francisco Nursing Department. (2001 November). Developmental needs of adults and ageing adults. *Peak Development for...Nursing Assistants, 4*(11), 1-2.

University of Michigan. (2006). *Population growth over human history.* Retrieved July 30, 2012, from http://www.globalchange.umich.edu/globalchange2/current/lectures/ human_pop/human_p...

Updike, J. (1991a). *The Rabbit omnibus.* Harmondsworth, UK: Penguin.

Updike, J. (1991b). *Rabbit at rest.* Harmondsworth, UK: Penguin.

Van der Reyden, D & Jourbert, R. (2005) HIV/AIDS in psychiatry: the moral and ethical dilemmas and issues facing occupational therapists treating persons with HIV/AIDS. In

R. Crouch, V. Alers (eds.) *Occupational therapy in psychiatry and mental health 4th ed.* (pp. 95-125). Chichester: Whurr.

Villamil, E., Huppert, F. A., & Melzer, D. (2006). Low prevalence of depression is linked to statutory retirement ages rather than a personal work exit: a national survey. *Psychological Medicine, 36(*7), 999-100.

Vincent, D. (1981). *Bread, knowledge and freedom, a study of nineteenth-century working class autobiography.* London: Europa Publications.

Walsh, S., Shulman, S., Feldman, B., & Maurer, O. (2005). The importance of immigration on the internal processes and developmental task of emerging. *Journal of Youth and Adolescence, 34*(5), 413-426.

Ward, M. (1988). *One camp chair in the living room.* Brighton, UK: QueenSpark.

wa Thiong'o, N. (1982). *Detained: A writer's prison diary.* Nairobi: Heinemann Educational Books.

Werskey, G. (1994). *The visible college. A collective biography of British scientists and socialists of the 1930s.* London: Free Association Books.

Wheway, E. (1984). *Edna's story, memories of life in a children's home and in service in Dorset and London.* Wimborne, UK: Words and Action.

White, H. R., & Jackson, K. (2008). Social and psychological influences on emerging adult drinking behavior [Electronic version]. *Social and Psychological Influences on Emerging Adult Drinking Behavior.* Retrieved May 20, 2008, from http://www.addictioninfo.org/articles/2254/1/Social-and-Psychological-Influences-on-Em...

Whiteford, G. (1997). Occupational deprivation and incarceration. *Journal of Occupational Science, 4*(3), 126-130.

Whiteford, G. (2000). Occupational deprivation: Global challenge in the new millennium. *British Journal of Occupational Therapy. 63*(5), 200-204.

Whiteford, G., & Townsend, E. (2011). Participatory occupational justice framework (POJF 2010): Enabling occupational participation and inclusion. In F. Kronenberg, N. Pollard, & D. Sakellariou (Eds), *Occupational therapies without borders* (Vol. 2, pp. 65-84). St. Louis, MO: Elsevier.

Whitmarsh, L., Seyfang, G., O'Neill, S. (2011). Public engagement with carbon and climate change: To what extent is the public 'carbon capable'? *Global Environmental Change* 21, 56–65.

Wick, G. (2010). Personal ideas on successful aging. *Gerontology, 56*(2), 121-122.

Wilcock, A. A. (2006). *An occupational perspective of health.* Thorofare, NJ: Slack Inc.

Wilding, C., & Whiteford. G. (2007) Occupation and occupational therapy: Knowledge paradigms and everyday practice. *Australian Occupational Therapy Journal, 54,* 185–193.

Wilcock, A. A. (2006). *An occupational perspective of health.* Thorofare, NJ: Slack.

Williams, R. (1976). *Keywords.* London: Fontana.

Wilson, D. S. (2002). *Darwin's cathedral: Evolution, religion, and the nature of society.* Chicago: University of Chicago Press.

Wilson, D. S. (2005). Testing major evolutionary hypotheses about religion with a random sample. *Human nature, 16*(4), 419-446.

Wilson, D. S. (2007). Evolution: One for all [Electronic version]. *American Scientist: Research Triangle Park, 95*, 269-271. Retrieved April 10, 2008, from http://proquest.umi.com/pqdweb?index=8&sid=4&srchmode=1&vinst=PROD&fmt=3&s t

Wilson, D. S., Van Vugt, M., & O'Gorman, R. (2008). Multilevel selection theory and major evolutionary transitions: Implications for psychological science. *Current Directions in Psychological Science, 17*(1), 6-9.

Wiltshire, P. (1985). *Living and winning.* Hackney, UK: Centerprise.

Winnicott, D. W. (1971). *Playing and reality.* London: Tavistock.

Winther, M. (2004). *The golden blackbird* [Electronic version]. Retrieved April 20, 2008, from http://home.swipnet.se/~w-73784/golden.htm.

Wolpert, L. (2007, Winter). *Interview with Lewis Wolpert. Science in School, 7*, 9-11.

Wolveridge, J. (1981). *Ain't it grand (or 'this was Stepney').* London: Journeyman.

Woodin, T. (2005). Muddying the waters: Changes in class and identity in a working class cultural organization. *Sociology, 39*, 1001-1018.

Woolley, T. (2009). *Earth's human carrying capacity.* Found at http://msemac.redwoods.edu/-darnold/math55/DEProj/sp09/TerranWoolley/Finalpaper.

World Health Organization. (2001). *International classification of functioning, disability and health.* Geneva, Switzerland: Author.

World Health Organization. (2002). *Active ageing: A policy framework.* Retrieved April 10, 2004, from http://www.who.int/hpr/ageing/ActiveAgeingPolicyFrame.pdf.

World Health Organization. (2003). *Climate change and human health – risks and responses.* Geneva, Switzerland: Author.

Worrall, B. G. (1988). *The making of the modern church. Christianity in England since 1800.* London: SPCK.

Wren, T. (1998). *Flying sparks.* Brighton, UK: QueenSpark.

Yerxa, E. J. (1967). Authentic occupational therapy. *American Journal of Occupational Therapy, 21*, 1-9.

Zeldin, T. (1979). *France 1848-1945: Ambition and Love.* Oxford: Oxford University Press.

Index

www.ingramcontent.com/pod-product-compliance
Lightning Source LLC
LaVergne TN
LVHW062209200926
848484LV00006B/1358